PAST AND PRESENT OF THE MEDITERRANEAN DIET

Revolutionize Your Kitchen Thanks To These Innovative Recipes Modeled On Mediterranean Principles.

Mediterranean Flavor

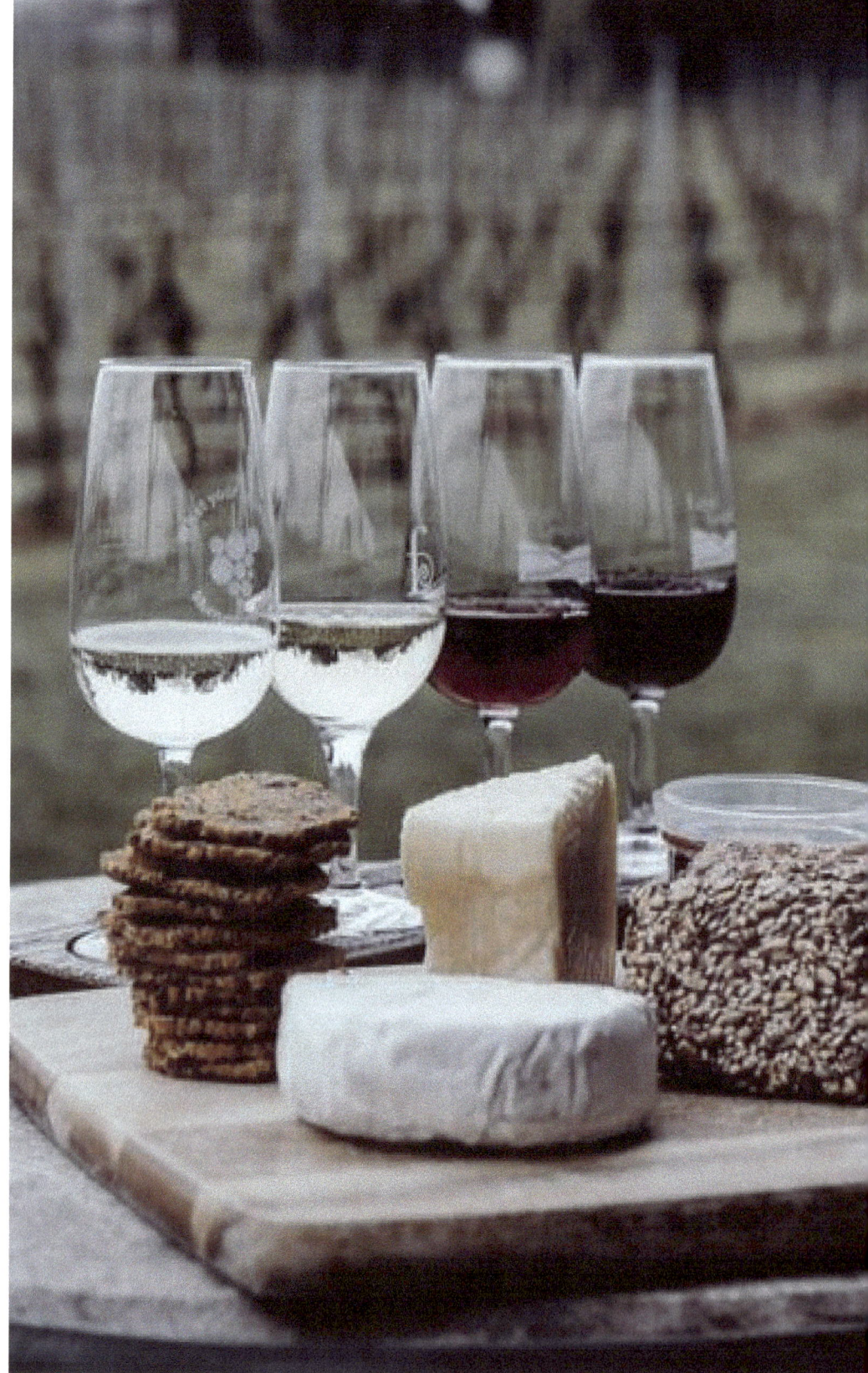

© Copyright 2020 by Mediterranean Flavor - All rights reserved.

The following Book is reproduced below to provide information that is as accurate and reliable as possible. Regardless, purchasing this Book can be seen as consent to the fact that both the publisher and the author of this book are in no way experts on the topics discussed within and that any recommendations or suggestions that are made herein are for entertainment purposes only. Professionals should be consulted as needed before undertaking any of the actions endorsed herein.

This declaration is deemed fair and valid by both the American Bar Association and the Committee of Publishers Association and is legally binding throughout the United States.

Furthermore, the transmission, duplication, or reproduction of any of the following work including specific information will be considered an illegal act irrespective of if it is done electronically or in print. This extends to creating a secondary or tertiary copy of the work or a recorded copy and is only allowed with the express written consent from the Publisher. All additional rights reserved.

The information in the following pages is broadly considered a truthful and accurate account of facts and as such, any inattention, use, or misuse of the information in question by the reader will render any resulting actions solely under their purview. There are no scenarios in which the publisher or the original author of this work can be in any fashion deemed liable for any hardship or damages that may befall them after undertaking the information described herein.

Additionally, the information in the following pages is intended only for informational purposes and should thus be thought of as universal. As befitting its nature, it is presented without assurance regarding its prolonged validity or interim quality. Trademarks that are mentioned are done without written consent and can in no way be considered an endorsement from the trademark holder.

Table of Contents

INTRODUCTION 1

BREAKFAST 18
- Zucchini with Quinoa Pan 19
- Spicy Peas Omelet 21
- Low Carb Smoothie 22
- Fig with Cheese Oatmeal 23
- Berries Pudding 25
- Walnuts Yogurt 26
- Egg-Feta Scramble 27
- Chickpeas Bowls 29
- Crispy Veggie Bowls 31
- Vanilla Flavored Oats 33

LUNCH 34
- Roasted Veggies with Brown Rice Bowl 36
- Rustic Lentil with Basmati Rice Pilaf 38
- Tasty Spanish Rice 40
- Tomato Chicken Pasta 43
- Black Bean Pasta with Shrimp 45
- Almond Butter Swoodles 47
- Black Bean Burgers and Brown Rice 50
- Falafel with Tahini 52
- Tangy Tomato Panini 54
- Chicken Wraps 56

- BRUNCH 58
  - Lemon Artichokes 60
  - Pepper Zucchinis 62
  - Tasty Okra 63
  - Cauliflower with Dill 64
  - Eggplant with Parsnips 67
  - Garlic Beans 68
  - Olives with Eggplant 69
  - Broccoli & Vegan Carrots 72
  - Seasonal Vegitable Ratatouille 74
  - Coconut Clam Chowder 76
- DINNER 78
  - Vegetable Stew 80
  - Classical Spinach & Feta Lasagna 81
  - Sage Flan and Green Beans 83
  - Grilled Cauliflower Steaks & Steamed Asparagus 86
  - Green Bell Pepper & Mushroom Stew 88
  - Traditional Spanish Pisto 90
  - Greek Salad with Dill Dressing 92
  - Zucchini Spaghetti and Avocado & Capers 95
  - Vegan Minestrone 96
  - Kale & Cauliflower Cheese Waffles 98
- DESSERT 100
  - Almond Rice 102

Frozen Strawberry Yogurt 103

Almond Peaches 104

Raisin Baked Apples 105

Walnuts Sweet Cake 106

Tasty Cookies 107

Cinnamon Cakes 109

Yummy Yogurt Cake 110

Apple Sauce with Chunks 112

Olives Cake 113

SALADS AND SOUPS 115

Pinto Bean Salad 117

Chicken Salad Pitas 120

Mulligatawny Soup 122

Ranch Chicken Soup 123

Classical Chicken Soup 126

Soothing Chicken Noodle Soup 128

Cabbage and Chicken Soup 130

Enchilada Soup 132

BBQ Chicken Pizza Soup 133

Grilled Salmon Soup 135

INTRODUCTION

The Mediterranean Diet is the traditional diet of the countries surrounding the Mediterranean Sea, such as Greece, Spain, and Italy. It focuses on the regional foods from those countries, which have many benefits, including improving heart health, chronic disease, and obesity.

The Mediterranean Diet reflects the personality of these regions and includes a wonderful variety of ingredients and recipes, featuring grains, fats from fish, olive oil, nuts, fruits, and lean meats. It is easy to follow and will provide lots of healthy and delicious meals that your family will love.

This diet is generally characterized by a high intake of plant-based food such as fresh fruits, vegetables, nuts and cereals, and olive oil, with a moderate amount of fish and poultry, and a small amount of dairy products, red meats, and sweets. Wine is allowed with every meal but at a moderate level. The Mediterranean Diet focuses strongly on social and cultural activities like communal mealtimes, resting after eating, and physical activities.

The Mediterranean Diet is not simply a weight loss or fad diet; however, raising your dietary fiber and cutting down on red meat, animal fats, and processed foods will lead to weight loss and a decreased risk of many diseases.

The Mediterranean Diet Pyramid

The Mediterranean Diet Pyramid is a visual tool that summarizes the diet. It suggests pattern of eating and gives guidelines for meal frequency and food management. This pyramid allows you to develop healthy eating habits and maintain calorie counts as well.

The pyramid tiers consist of the following groups:

- **Plant-based foods**

This includes olive oil, fruits, vegetables, whole grains, legumes, beans, nuts and seeds, and spices and herbs. These foods should be part of every meal. Olive oil is the main fat used in cooking. It can occasionally be replaced with butter or cooking oil, but in smaller quantities.

Fresh herbs and spices can be used in generous amounts in dishes for enhancing taste and as an alternative to salt. Dried herbs can also be used. Fresh ginger and garlic are always allowed for flavor.

- **Seafood**

Seafood is an important staple and one of the main sources of protein in the Mediterranean Diet. Make sure you have seafood at least twice a week. There are many varieties of fish that will work, as well as mussels, shrimps, and crab. Tuna is a great source of protein and works well in sandwiches and salads.

- **Dairy and Poultry**

Yogurt, milk, cheese, and poultry can be consumed ata moderate level. If you use eggs in cooking and baking, include them in your weekly limit. Choose healthy cheese options like ricotta, feta, and Parmesan. You can have them as toppings and garnishing your meals and dishes.

- **Sweets and Red Meat**

Sweets and meats are used less in this diet. If you eat them, cut down on the quantity and choose lean meat. Red meat, sugar, and fat are not good for heart health and blood sugar.

- **Water**

The Mediterranean Diet encourages increased daily water intake, 9 8-ounce glasses for women and 13 for men. For pregnant and breastfeeding women, the amount should be higher.

- **Wine**

The Mediterranean Diet allows for moderate wine consumption with meals. Alcohol reduces the risk of heart disease. One glass of wine for women and two for men is the recommended daily limit.

Foods That Are Not Allowed in the Mediterranean Diet

This diet satisfies your food cravings by providing better alternatives. It helps you to shift your mindset from looking for snacks to having fresh fruits and vegetables that will satisfy your between-meal hunger.

The following items should be restricted or replaced by healthy options:

- **Added sugar**

Sugar is one of the most difficult items to avoid in your diet. Try to stick to healthy sugar from fresh fruits and vegetables. Avoid processed foods; the added sugars in pasta sauce, peanut butter, fruit juices, bread, and bakery products are considered empty calories.

Added sugars are commonly used in processed food like:

- High fructose corn syrup
- Glucose
- Corn syrup

- Sucrose
- Maltose
- Corn sweetener

You can add fresh fruits like strawberries and raspberries to your water for flavor and refreshment as well as eating them. Switch to an organic sweetener like honey or maple syrup instead of using refined sugars.

- **Refined grains**

Refined grains are prohibited in the Mediterranean Diet because they lead to heart disease and type 2 diabetes. Grains are often grouped with carbohydrates, but they do not fall into the "bad carbs" category until they are refined. Refined grains go through a milling process during which the major nutrients are removed. They are left with less fiber, iron, and vitamins and more empty calories.

The most common refined grains consist of:

- White flour
- White bread
- White rice
- White flour pizza crust

- **Breakfast cereals**

Whole grains are a better alternative. When possible, choose sourdough bread. Enjoy sandwiches in a whole-grain wrap or pita bread. You can also try plant-based alternatives like cauliflower crust, cauliflower rice, or spiralized vegetables in place of pasta. Swap in whole grains like quinoa and brown rice.

- **Refined Oils**

Refined oils are extremely damaging to your health. The key nutrients have been stripped from out and additional chemicals added in, making their way to your food.

Most oils are extracted from the seeds of plants. This includes soybean oil, corn oil, sunflower oil, peanut oil, and olive oil. Vegetable oils are a combination of multiple plants. The process of extracting the oil involves a variety of chemicals that can increase inflammation in the body. The fat that remains in the oil has been linked to several health conditions such as cancer, heart disease, and diabetes. Oils are also used to create margarine in a hydrogenation process, using chemicals that allow the oil to remain in a solid-state. When the oil is hydrogenated, the fatty acids that were in the oil are further destroyed and transformed into trans fatty acids. Several scientific studies have been conducted to show the connection of trans fatty acids to some debilitating health conditions.

Trans fatty acids are considered to be some of the unhealthiest fats you can consume, especially when it comes to your heart. These industrially manufactured fats cause LDL cholesterol to increase. High amounts of LDL or bad cholesterol can clog and destroy your arteries and increase blood pressure. This significantly increases your risk of heart attack and stroke.

Some of the most common trans fats or hydrogenated oils that you might not be aware of include:

- Microwaveable popcorn
- Butter
- Margarine
- Vegetable oil
- Fried foods
- Pre-packaged muffins, cakes, doughnuts, and pastries
- Coffee creamers
- Prepared pizza dough or pizza crust
- Cake frosting
- Potato chips
- Crackers

The Mediterranean Diet focuses on replacing these refined oils and processed foods with more wholesome and natural ingredients. Refined oils can be easy to eliminate from your diet. If you are used to sautéing your foods with refined oil, switch to unrefined olive oil. Instead of frying foods in oil, bake or grill them.

- **Processed Meat**

Processed meats have been processed extensively to preserve flavors and provide a longer shelf life. The most common forms are bacon, hot dogs, deli meats, sausage, and canned meats. Consuming processed meat daily can cause or increase the risk of colorectal cancer, stomach cancer, pancreatic cancer, and prostate cancer.

Sodium is what makes processed meats so harmful. Sodium is well known to increase blood pressure, which increases the risk of different heart diseases. Processed meat contains at least 50 percent more preservatives than unprocessed meats. These preservatives affect sugar tolerances and can cause insulin resistance, which can lead to diabetes.

- Switch out processed meats and red meats for fish or poultry.
- Use vegetables or beans in place of meat.

- Use a variety of spices to add more flavor to a dish where you would use meat in the same way.
- Spices like cumin, coriander, peppercorn, and marjoram add unique flavors to the dish so you won't miss the bacon, sausage, or ground meat.
- You can use different seasonings on sautéed or baked vegetables.
- Add roasted chickpeas or toasted seeds and nuts to dishes for more texture. These can be great alternatives to dishes that call for bacon crumbles.

Common Mistakes in the Mediterranean Diet:

When you start a new diet, you will make some mistakes or encounter situations in which you don't know what to do. Before you get on the Mediterranean Diet plan, here is a heads-up about common mistakes that people make. If you know about these mistakes, you can avoid them and achieve success more quickly.

- **All or Nothing**

Your attitude toward your diet matters a lot. This is why you must make sure you are mentally prepared for it. It will be different from your ordinary lifestyle, which is why you need an abundance of information. To learn the benefits of this diet, you can ask the experts or people who have experienced it.

- **Eating the Same Things**

Don't eat the same things over and over again, day after day. One of the most common mistakes people make is that they think that eating the same kind of vegetables all week long will help them lose weight. You must have variety in your diet. The Mediterranean Diet allows you to have multiple kinds of dishes throughout the week, but maintain portion control.

- **Deprivation**

Another mistake people make is thinking that deprivation is the only way to lose weight. The main point of this diet plan is to give you energy while helping you lose weight. Deprivation will only make you weaker. This diet plan won't work if you don't eat at all, so be sure to keep this in mind.

- **Giving up**

Don't give up in the middle of the Mediterranean Diet. If you see yourself losing weight and you think, *now I can cheat a little* … resist. Since you've put so much effort into it already, don't give up now. If you have chocolate cravings, find a healthy alternative. It's easier to develop self-control if you can see the results, so keep your goals in mind and stay strong. Our bodies need time to adjust and stabilize in terms of the food we eat, so switching back and forth is never a good option.

- **Not setting goals**

One of the main mistakes people make is not setting goals when they start the diet. You must have a goal in terms of how much weight you want to lose and work toward it. When you don't have a plan, you will become distracted and be unable to reach your destination, no matter how hard you try.

- **Following the wrong plan**

Another common mistake is that you don't have enough knowledge about the plan you are following to lose weight. Maybe you are following the wrong plan, one that doesn't seem to work for you. If you're confused, don't decide by yourself to follow the Mediterranean Diet; consult an expert who can advise you on what to eat and do to adopt a healthy lifestyle. Many people try to keep their old habits while mixing in elements of the Mediterranean Diet, but if you don't follow the diet, you won't achieve the optimal results. Decide if you're willing to do it, and then do it right.

Your Mediterranean Shopping Guide

Apart from knowing how to start your diet, it is necessary to know a little about how to set-up your food charts.

What to have:

- Fresh vegetables: tomatoes, kale, spinach, cauliflower, Brussels sprouts, cucumbers, etc.
- Fresh fruits: An orange, apples, pears, grapes, dates, strawberries, figs, peaches, etc.
- Seeds and nuts: almonds, walnuts, cashews, sunflower seeds, etc.
- Legumes: beans, lentils, chickpeas, etc.
- Roots: yams, turnips, sweet potatoes, etc.
- Whole grains: whole oats, rye, brown rice, corn, barley, buckwheat, whole wheat, whole grain pasta, and bread
- Fish and seafood: sardines, salmon, tuna, shrimp, mackerel, oyster, crab, clams, mussels, etc.
- Poultry: turkey, chicken, duck, etc.
- Eggs—chicken, duck, quail
- Dairy products such as cheese, Greek yogurt, etc.

- Herbs and spices: mint, basil, garlic, rosemary, cinnamon, sage, pepper, etc.
- Healthy fats and oil: extra virgin olive oil, avocado oil, olives, etc.

What to avoid:

- Foods with added sugar like soda, ice cream, candy, table sugar, etc.
- Refined grains like white bread or pasta made with refined wheat
- Margarine and similar processed foods that contain trans fats
- Refined oil such as cottonseed oil, soybean oil, etc.
- Processed meat such as hot dogs, sausages, bacon, etc.
- Highly processed food with labels such as "Low-Fat" or "Diet," or anything that is not natural

Useful Information about Healthy Foods

1. **Oils**

The Mediterranean Diet emphasizes healthy oils. The following are some of the oils that you might want to consider.

- **Coconut oil:** Coconut oil is semi-solid at room temperature and can be used for months without turning sour. Coconut oil also has a lot of health benefits as lauric acid, which can help to improve cholesterol levels and kill various pathogens.

- **Extra-virgin olive oil:** Olive oil is well-known worldwide as one of the healthiest oils, and it is a key ingredient in the Mediterranean Diet. Olive oil can help to improve health biomarkers such as increasing HDL cholesterol and lowering the amount of bad LDL cholesterol.
- **Avocado oil:** Avocado oil is very similar to olive oil and has similar health benefits. It can be used for many purposes as an alternative to olive oil (such as in cooking).

2. **Healthy salt alternatives and spices**

Aside from replacing healthy oils, the Mediterranean Diet will allow you to opt for healthy salt alternatives as well.

- **Sunflower seeds**

Sunflower seeds are excellent and give a nutty and sweet flavor.

- **Fresh squeezed lemon**

Lemon is packed with Vitamin C, which helps to neutralize damaging free radicals from the system.

- **Onion powder**

Onion powder is a dehydrated ground spice made from an onion bulb, which is mostly used as a seasoning and is a fine salt alternative.

- **Black pepper**

Black pepper is also a salt alternative that is native to India. It is made by grinding whole peppercorns.

- **Cinnamon**

Cinnamon is well-known as a savory spice and available in two varieties: Ceylon and Chinese. Both of them sport a sharp, warm, and sweet flavor.

- **Fruit-infused vinegar**

Fruit-infused vinegar or flavored vinegar can give a nice flavor to meals. These are excellent ingredients to add a bit of flavor to meals without salt.

Eating Out on the Mediterranean Diet

It might seem a bit confusing, but eating out at a restaurant while on a Mediterranean Diet is pretty easy. Just follow the simple rules below:

- Try to ensure that you choose seafood or fish as the main dish of your meal
- When ordering, try to make a special request and ask the restaurant to fry their food using extra virgin olive oil
- Ask for only whole-grain based ingredients if possible
- If possible, try to read the menu before going to the restaurant
- Try to have a simple snack before you go out; this will help prevent you from overeating.

BREAKFAST

Zucchini with Quinoa Pan

6 Servings

Preparation Time: 20 minutes

Ingredients

- 1½ tomatoes, cubed
- 1 cup feta cheese, crumbled
- 3 cups water
- 1½ cups canned garbanzo beans, drained and rinsed
- A pinch of salt and black pepper
- 1½ tablespoons olive oil
- 2½ garlic cloves, minced
- 1½ cups quinoa
- 1½ zucchinis, roughly cubed
- 2½ tablespoons basil, chopped
- 1 cup green olives, pitted and chopped

Directions

- Heat up a pan with the oil over medium-high heat, add the garlic and quinoa, and brown for 3 minutes.
- Add in the water, zucchinis, salt, and pepper, toss, bring to a simmer and cook for 15 minutes.
- Add the rest of the ingredients, mix and divide everything between plates and serve for breakfast.

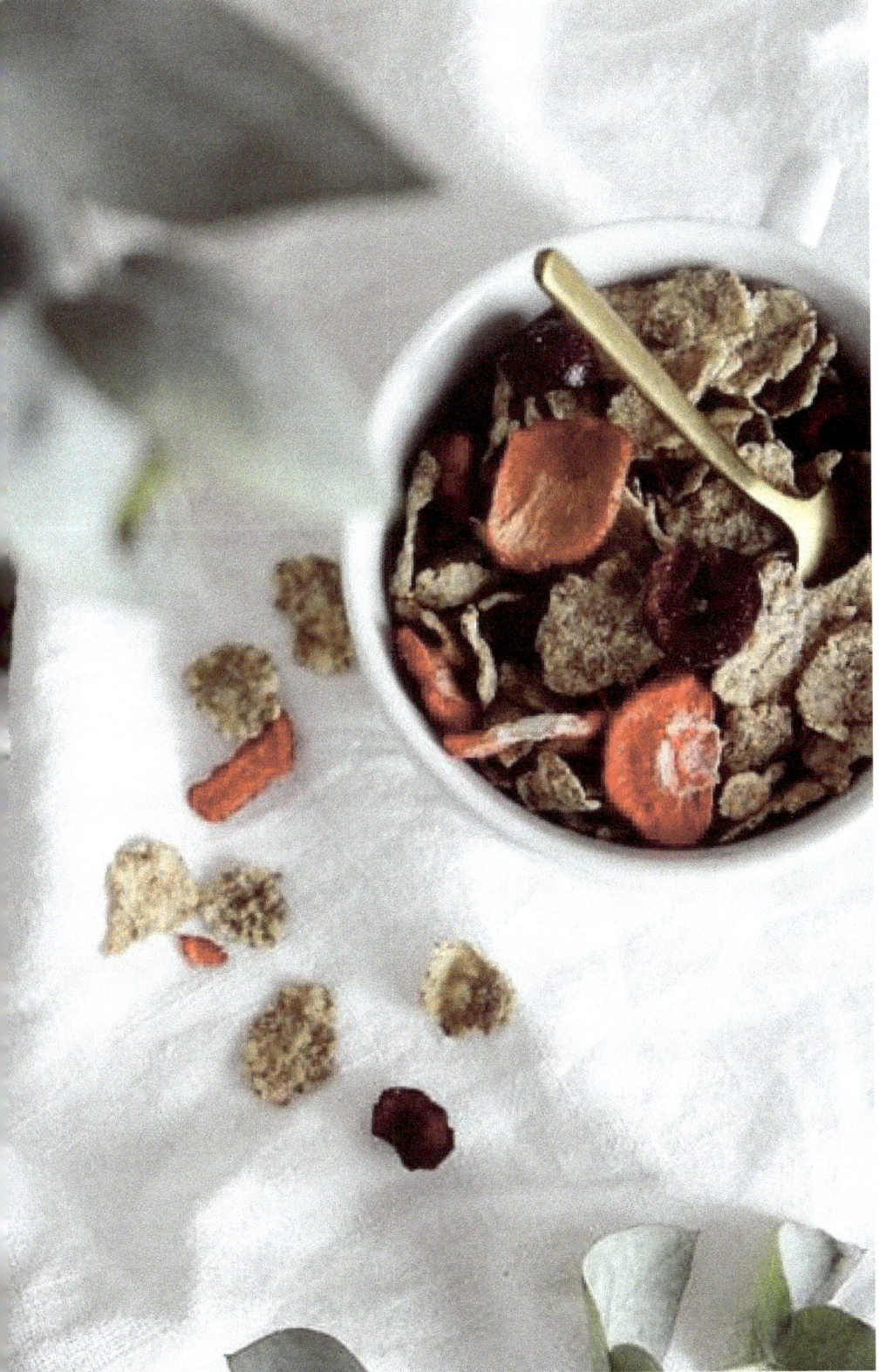

Spicy Peas Omelet

8 Servings

Preparation Time: 20 minutes

Ingredients

- 6 oz green peas
- 1 cup corn kernels
- 8 eggs, beaten
- 1 cup heavy cream
- 1 teaspoon of sea salt
- 1½ red bell peppers, chopped
- 1½ teaspoons butter

Directions

- Toss butter in the skillet and melt it.
- Add green peas, bell pepper, and corn kernels. Start to fry the vegetables over medium heat.
- In the mixing bowl, whisk together eggs, heavy cream, sea salt, and paprika.
- Pour the mixture over the roasted vegetables and stir well immediately.
- Close the lid and cook the omelet over medium-low heat for 15 minutes or until it is solid.
- Transfer the cooked omelet into the big plate and cut it into the servings.

Low Carb Smoothie

4 Servings

Preparation Time: 15 minutes

Ingredients

- 1 cup romaine lettuce
- 1 tablespoon fresh ginger, peeled and chopped
- 2 cups of filtered water
- 1/10 cup fresh pineapple, chopped
- 4 tablespoons fresh parsley
- 1 cup raw cucumber, peeled and sliced
- 1 Hass avocado
- 1 cup kiwi fruit, peeled and chopped

Directions

- Put all the ingredients in a blender and blend until smooth.
- Pour into 2 serving glasses and serve chilled.

Fig with Cheese Oatmeal

2 Servings

Preparation Time: 5 minutes

Ingredients

- 1 cup old-fashioned rolled oats
- 1½ tablespoons of almonds, toasted, sliced
- 1½ cups of water
- Pinch of salt
- 3 teaspoons honey
- 3 tablespoons ricotta cheese, part-skim
- 3 tablespoons dried figs, chopped

Directions

- Pour the water into a small saucepan and add the salt; bring to a boil.
- Stir in the oats and reduce heat to medium. Cook the oats for about 5 minutes, occasionally stirring, until most of the water is absorbed.
- Remove the pan from the heat, cover, and let stand for 2-3 minutes.
- Serve topped with the figs, almonds, ricotta, and drizzle of honey.

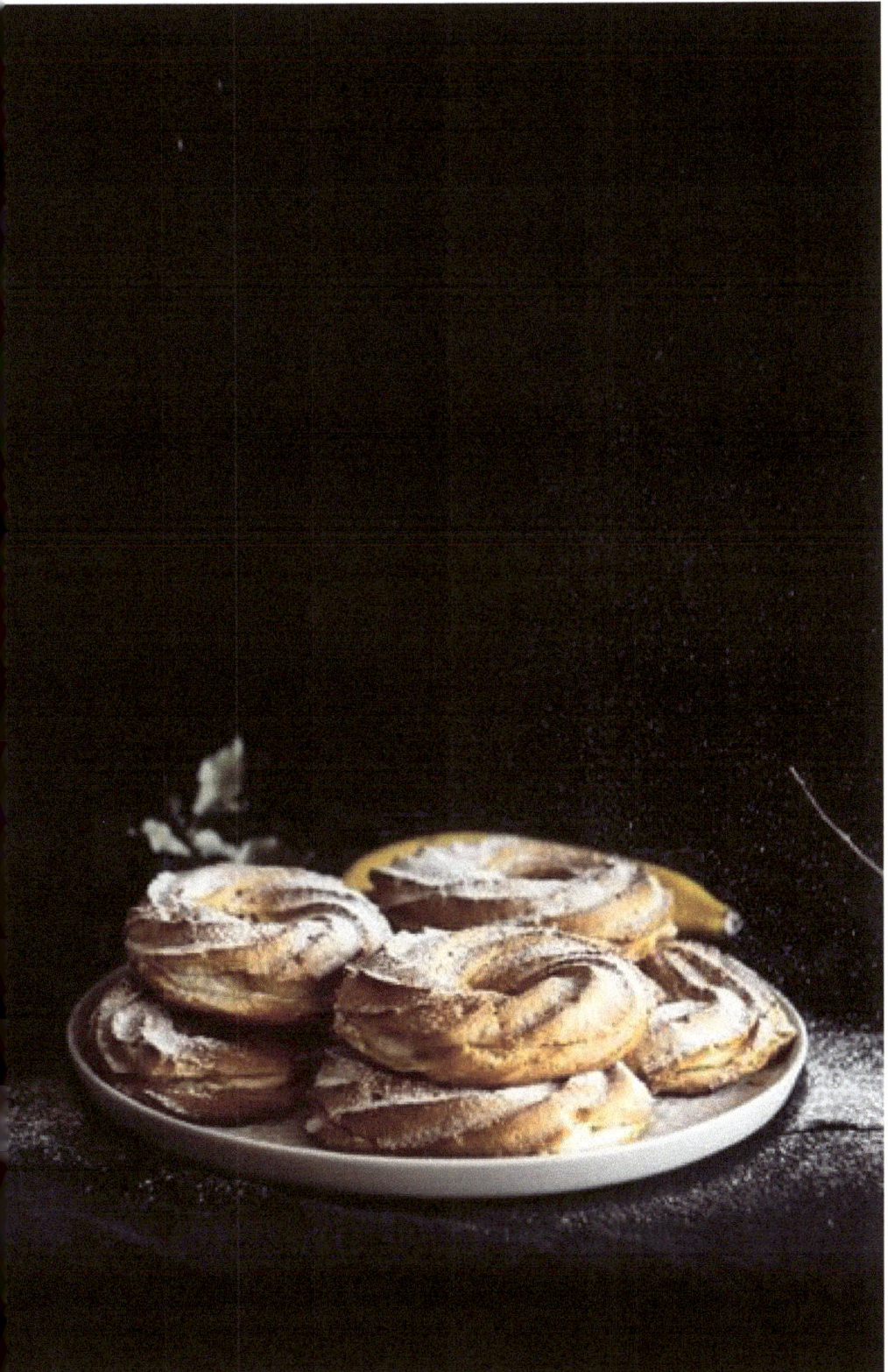

Berries Pudding

4 Servings

Preparation Time: 30 minutes

Ingredients

- 1 cup raspberries
- 2½ teaspoons maple syrup
- 2 cups of plain yogurt
- 1 teaspoon ground cardamom
- 1 cup of chia seeds, dried

Directions

- Mix up together Plain yogurt with maple syrup and ground cardamom.
- Add Chia seeds. Stir it gently.
- Put the yogurt in the serving glasses and top with the raspberries.
- Refrigerate the breakfast for at least 30 minutes or overnight.

Walnuts Yogurt

6 Servings

Preparation Time: 5 minutes

Ingredients

- 3 cups Greek yogurt
- 2 cups walnuts, chopped
- 1½ teaspoons vanilla extract
- 1 cup honey
- 2 teaspoons cinnamon powder

Directions

- In a bowl, combine the yogurt with the walnuts and the rest of the ingredients, toss, divide into smaller bowls and keep in the fridge for 10 minutes before serving for breakfast

Egg-Feta Scramble

6 Servings

Preparation Time: 15 minutes

Ingredients

- 1 teaspoon dry oregano
- 1 teaspoon dry basil
- 1½ teaspoons of olive oil
- A few cracks freshly ground black pepper
- Warm whole-wheat tortillas, optional
- 8 eggs
- 3 cups crumbled feta cheese
- 2½ tablespoons green onions, minced
- 2½ tablespoons red peppers, roasted, diced
- 1 teaspoon kosher salt
- 1 teaspoon garlic powder
- 1 cup Greek yogurt

Directions

- Preheat a pan over medium heat.
- In a bowl, whisk the eggs, sour cream, basil, oregano, garlic powder, salt, and pepper. Gently add the feta.

- When the skillet is hot, add the olive oil and then the egg mixture; allow the egg mix to set, then scrape the bottom of the pan to let the uncooked egg cook. Stir in the red peppers and the green onions. Continue cooking until the egg mixture is cooked to your preferred doneness. Serve immediately.

Chickpeas Bowls

6 Servings

Preparation Time: 30 minutes

Ingredients

- 1½ teaspoons coriander, ground
- 1½ tablespoons olive oil
- A pinch of salt and black pepper
- 1 cup Greek yogurt
- 1 cup green olives, pitted and halved
- 17 ounces canned chickpeas, drained and rinsed
- 1 teaspoon cardamom, ground
- 1 teaspoon cinnamon powder
- 2 teaspoons turmeric powder
- 1 cup cherry tomatoes, halved
- 1½ cucumbers, sliced

Directions

- Spread the chickpeas on a lined baking sheet, add the cardamom, cinnamon, turmeric, coriander, oil, salt, and pepper, toss and bake at 375 degrees F for 30 minutes.
- In a bowl, combine the roasted chickpeas with the rest of the ingredients, toss and serve for breakfast.

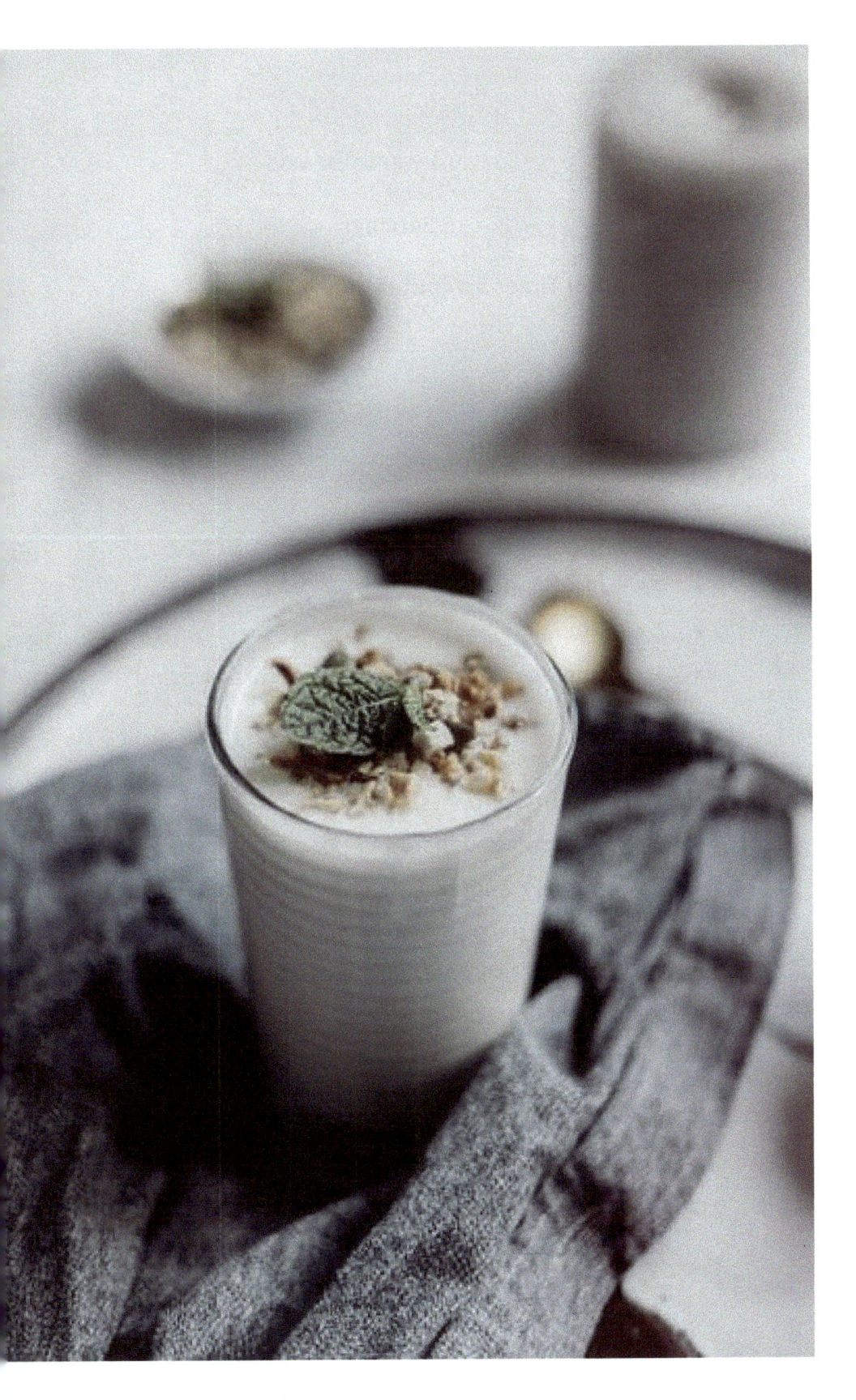

Crispy Veggie Bowls

6 Servings

Preparation Time: 5 minutes

Ingredients

- 1½ red onions, chopped
- 1½ cups mint, chopped
- 3 cups feta cheese, crumbled
- 2½ tablespoons olive oil
- 3 cups whole-wheat orzo, cooked
- 16 ounces canned cannellini beans, drained and rinsed
- 1½ yellow bell peppers, cubed
- 1½ green bell peppers, cubed
- A pinch of salt and black pepper
- 3½ tomatoes, cubed
- 1 cup lemon juice
- 1½ tablespoons lemon zest, grated
- 1½ cucumbers, cubed
- 2 cups kalamata olives, pitted and sliced
- 3½ garlic cloves, minced

Directions

- In a salad bowl, combine the orzo with the beans, bell peppers, and the rest of the ingredients, toss, divide the mix between plates and serve for breakfast.

Vanilla Flavored Oats

6 Servings

Preparation Time: 10 minutes

Ingredients

- 3 teaspoons of honey
- 3 tablespoons Plain yogurt
- 1 cup rolled oats
- 1½ cups of milk
- 1½ teaspoons vanilla extract
- 1½ teaspoons ground cinnamon
- 1½ teaspoons butter

Directions

- Pour milk into the saucepan and bring it to boil.
- Add rolled oats and stir well.
- Close the lid and simmer the oats for 5 minutes over medium heat. The cooked oats will absorb all milk.
- Then add butter and stir the oats well.
- In the separated bowl, whisk together Plain yogurt with honey, cinnamon, and vanilla extract.
- Transfer the cooked oats into the serving bowls.
- Top the oats with the yogurt mixture in the shape of the wheel.

LUNCH

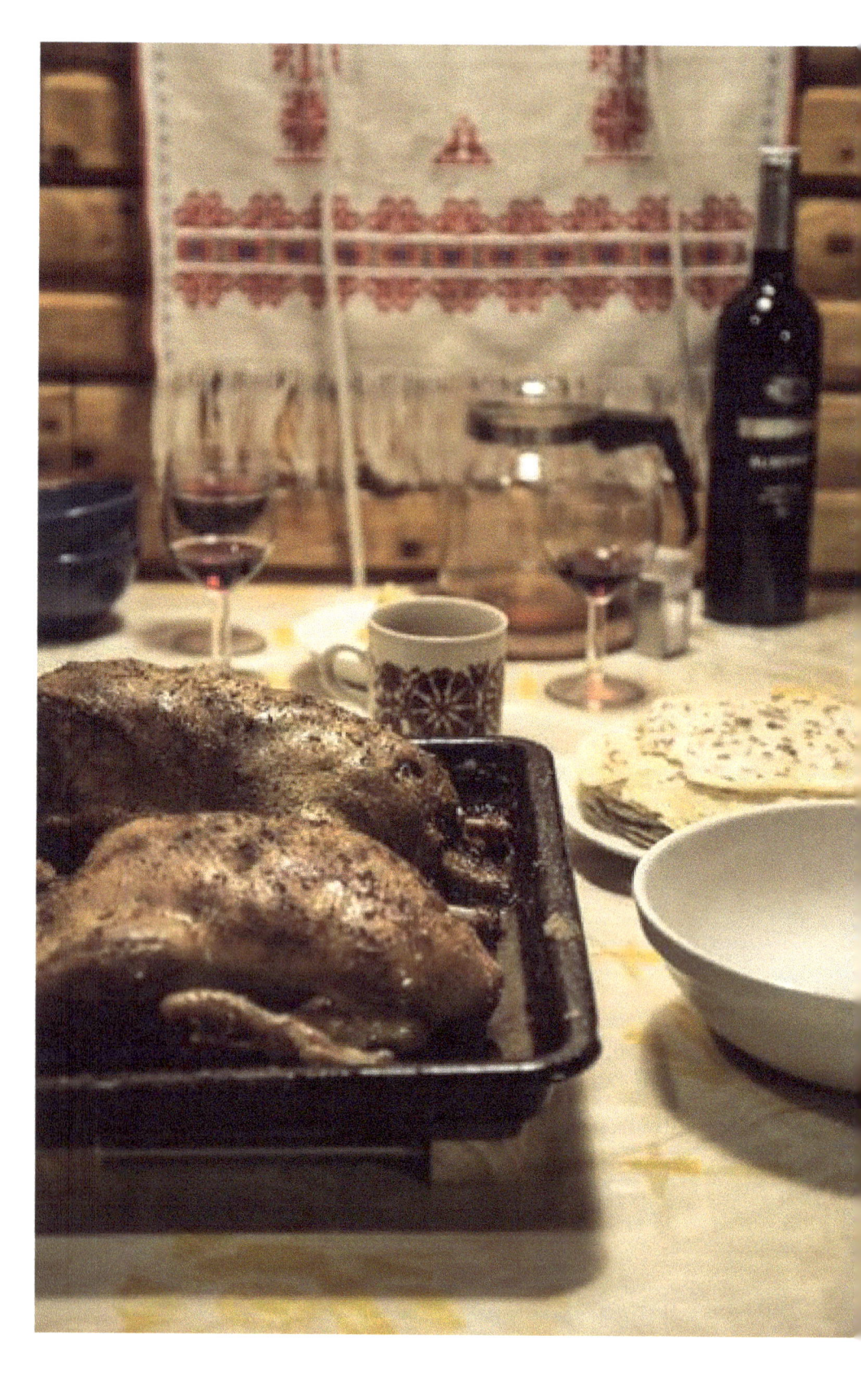

Roasted Veggies with Brown Rice Bowl

6 Servings

Preparation Time: 45 minutes

Ingredients

Veggies and grains:

- 2½ cups cooked chickpeas or 1 can, rinsed and drained.
- 2½ tbsps sesame seeds.
- 2½ tsps extra virgin olive oil.
- Salt/pepper.
- 1½ head cauliflower, cut into bite-size pieces.
- 1½ head broccoli, cut into bite-size pieces.
- 3 ½ medium carrots, cut into coins.
- 1½ cups brown rice, i nearly always use quick-cook brown rice.

Creamy sweet tahini dressing:

- 1½ garlic cloves (minced).
- 3½ tbsps of nutritional yeast.
- ¼ cup water (plus more as needed to thin).
- Salt/pepper to taste.
- ¼ cups tahini.
- 3 tbsps balsamic vinegar.
- 2 tbsps pure maple syrup.

Directions

- Preheat oven to 400° F.
- Cook the rice according to package directions.
- Spread the cauliflower and broccoli on one baking sheet. Place the chickpeas and carrots on another baking sheet. Sprinkle 1 tsp oil over each baking sheet and give veggies and mix it. Sprinkle with salt and pepper.
- Roast for about 20-30 minutes, turning the pans and giving them a shake every ten minutes. Cauliflower and broccoli take about 30 minutes, carrots and chickpeas take about 20, so first add the broccoli/cauliflower and then add chickpeas/carrots after 10 minutes.
- Combine all the dressing ingredients in a small bowl and mix until smooth. Add more water, as needed, to thin. Set aside.
- When veggies and chickpeas are done, Add a little rice, broccoli, cauliflower, carrots, chickpeas, sesame seeds, and dressing in each bowl.

Rustic Lentil with Basmati Rice Pilaf

8 Servings

Preparation Time: 55 minutes

Ingredients

- 1½ teaspoons salt.
- 6 cups water.
- 2½ cups brown lentils, picked over and rinsed.
- 1½ cups basmati rice.
- 1 cup olive oil.
- 1½ large onions, chopped.
- 1½ teaspoons ground cumin.

Directions

- Warm the olive oil in a saucepan over medium heat. Add in the onions and cook for about 4 minutes until the onions are golden in color.
- Add the cumin, salt, and water on high heat. Boil the mixture for about 3 minutes.

- Lower the heat to medium-low and add the brown lentils. Simmer it for about 20 minutes until tender.
- Add in the basmati rice and stir well. Cook for about 20 minutes until the rice has absorbed the liquid completely.
- Using a fork to fluff the rice, cover, and let stand for 5 minutes.
- Transfer to plates and serve hot.

Tasty Spanish Rice

6 Servings

Preparation Time: 25 minutes

Ingredients

- 1½ teaspoons smoked paprika.
- 2½ tablespoons tomato paste.
- 1½ cups basmati rice.
- 1½ teaspoons of salt.
- 2½ tablespoons olive oil.
- 1½ medium onions, finely chopped.
- 1½ large tomatoes, finely diced.
- 3½ cups water.

Directions

- Warm the olive oil in a saucepan over medium heat. Add in the onions and tomato and cook for about 3 minutes until softened.
- Add in the paprika, tomato paste, basmati rice, and salt. Mix the mixture for 1 minute and slowly pour in the water.
- Lower the heat and allow simmering covered for about 12 minutes, stirring it constantly.

- Remove from the heat and let it rest in the saucepan for about 3 minutes.
- Serve the rice in the four serving bowls.

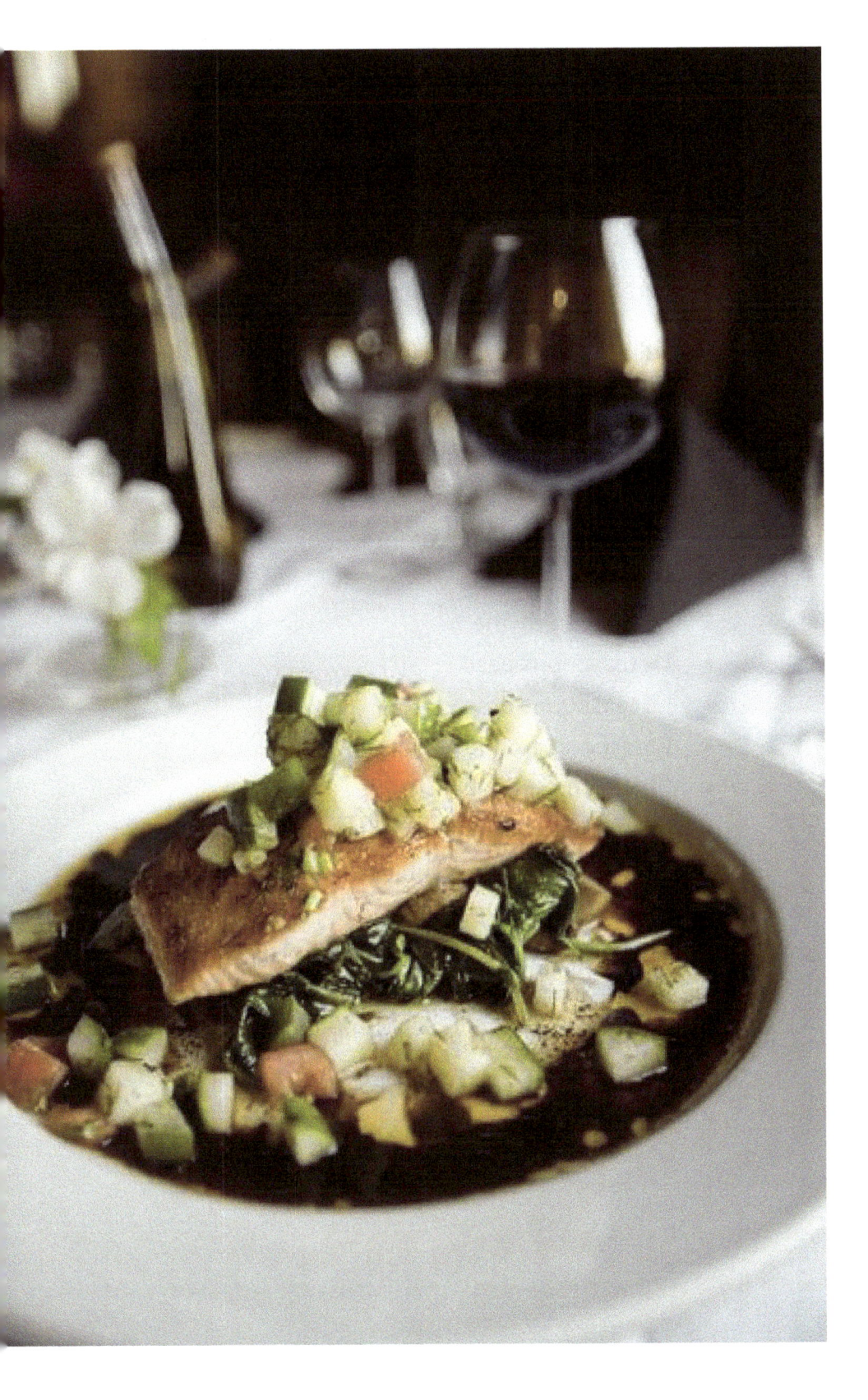

Tomato Chicken Pasta

6 Servings

Preparation Time: 3 hr 20 minutes

Ingredients

- 2 cups low-sodium chicken broth.
- 1½ stalk celeries, finely chopped.
- 1½ medium onions, cut into wedges.
- 1 teaspoon rosemary.
- 1 teaspoon thyme.
- 1½ teaspoons basil.
- 1½ teaspoons oregano.
- 1 teaspoon ground cinnamon.
- 1 teaspoon sea salt.
- 1 cup uncooked medium shell pasta.
- 1 cup feta cheese crumbled.
- 3 tablespoons olive oil.
- 1 pound (454 g) boneless, skinless chicken breasts, cut into 1-inch cubes.
- 15 ounces (425 g) tomatoes, diced.
- 2 medium carrots thinly sliced.
- 1½ cups freshly squeezed tomato juice.

Directions

- Add 2 tablespoons of olive oil into a slow cooker.
- Warm the remaining olive oil in a nonstick pan over medium-high heat.
- Add in the chicken to the pan and cook for about 6 minutes until lightly browned on all sides.
- Remove the chicken to a plate, and pat dry with paper towels, then move them into the slow cooker.
- Add in the tomatoes, carrots, tomato juice, chicken stock, celery, and onion to the slow cooker, then spice with rosemary, thyme, basil, oregano, cinnamon, and salt. Stir to mix well.
- Put the slow cooker lid on and cook on high for about 2 hours and 30 minutes.
- Add the pasta to the slow cooker. Place the lid on and cook for an additional 40 minutes or until the pasta is al dente.
- Serve the pasta, chicken, and vegetables on a large plate, and spread the feta cheese on top before serving.

Black Bean Pasta with Shrimp

6 Servings

Preparation Time: 25 minutes

Ingredients

- 4 tablespoons olive oil.
- 3 garlic cloves, minced.
- 1 onion, finely chopped.
- 1 pound (454 g) fresh shrimp, peeled and deveined.
- Salt and pepper, to taste.
- ¾ cup low-sodium chicken broth.
- 1 package black bean pasta.
- ¼ cup basil cut into strips.

Directions

- Put the black bean pasta in a large pot of boiling water and cook for about 6 minutes.
- Remove the pasta from the heat. Strain and rinse with cold water, then set the pasta aside on a platter.
- Warm olive oil in a large pan over medium heat. Add the garlic and onion, and then cook for 3 minutes until the onion is translucent.

- Add the shrimp and season with salt and pepper. Cook for 3 minutes, stirring occasionally, or until the shrimp is opaque. Pour in the chicken broth and let it simmer for 2 to 3 minutes until heated through.
- Remove the shrimp from the heat to the platter of pasta. Pour the liquid over the pasta and garnish with basil, and then serve.

Almond Butter Swoodles

6 Servings

Preparation Time: 1 hr 5 minutes

Ingredients

- 1½ tablespoons fresh lemon juice.
- 1½ tablespoons honey.
- 1 ½teaspoons paprika.
- 1/8 teaspoon ground red pepper (optional).
- Sea salt and ground black pepper.
- 1/4 cup water.
- 1/4 cup chopped yellow onion.
- 1-inch piece fresh ginger, peeled and sliced.
- 1 garlic clove.
- 3/4 cup almond butter.
- 1 tablespoon tamari.

For Swoodles:
- Sweet potatoes, spiralized (tool).
- 1/4 cup organic virgin coconut oil, melted.
- Sea salt and ground black pepper.

For Serving:

- ½ cup thinly sliced scallions.
- ½ cup fresh parsley, chopped.

- Simple cashew slaw.

Directions

- Preheat the oven to 425°F. Line the rimmed baking sheet with parchment paper.
- Make the sauce: In a blender, combine the onion, ginger, and garlic and pulse a few times until finely chopped. Add in the almond butter, tamari, lemon juice, honey, paprika, ground red pepper, and salt and black pepper to taste. Blend until combined. Stop to scrape down the sides.
- Pour the water through the feed hole. Keep blending until thick and creamy.
- Make the swoodles: Mix the sweet potatoes with the oil, making sure the pieces are well coated in a medium bowl. Place on the prepared baking sheet. Season with salt and black pepper. Bake for about 20 minutes. Check for doneness around the 10-minute mark, and check again periodically, to remove any swoodles that have cooked more quickly than the others.
- Serve the swoodles between 4 plates. Add a little of the sauce, 1 tablespoon scallions, and 1 tablespoon parsley on the top. Serve immediately with a vegan cashew slaw on the side.

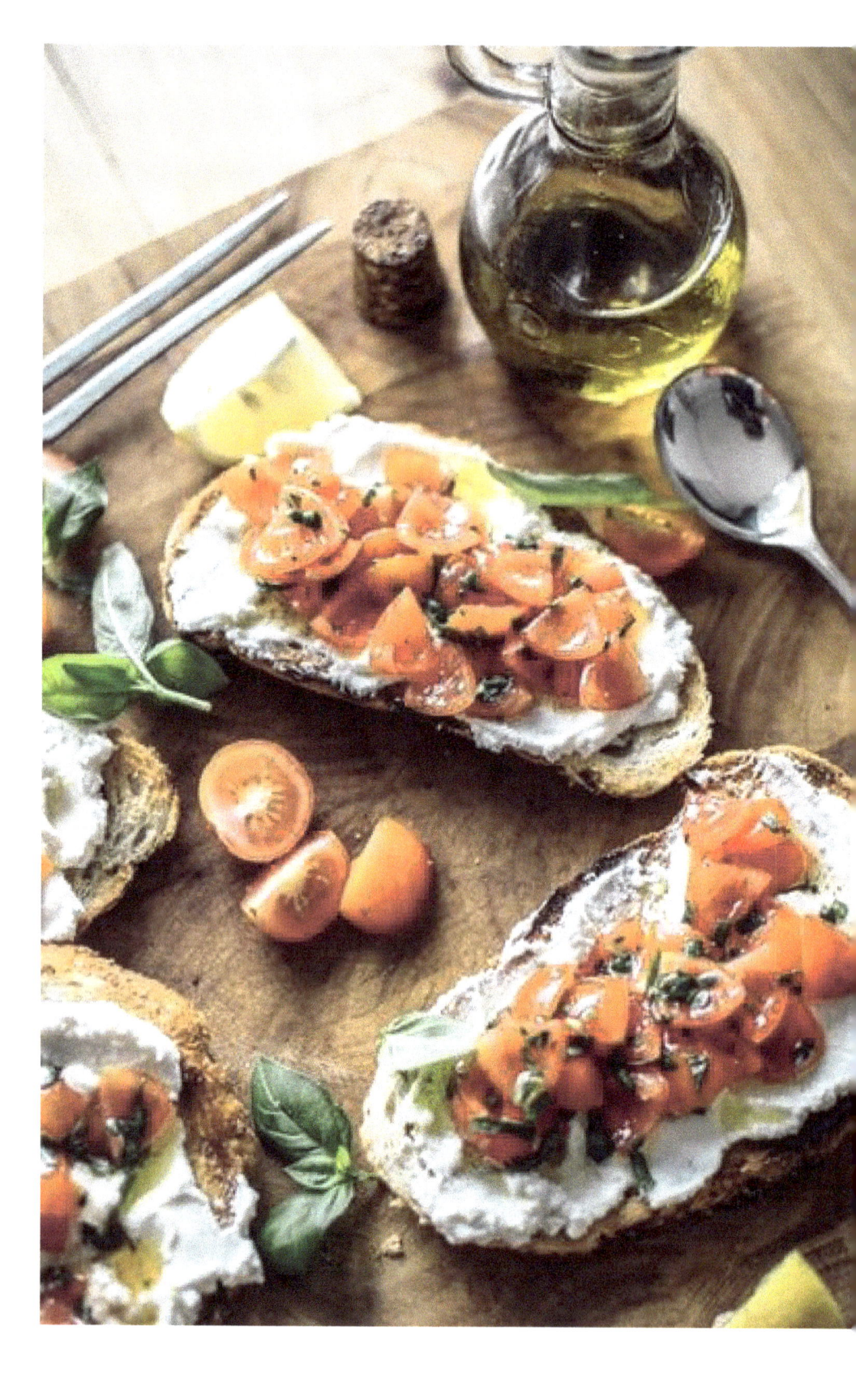

Black Bean Burgers and Brown Rice

6 Servings

Preparation Time: 40 minutes

Ingredients

- 1½ cups frozen corn.
- 1½ teaspoons salt.
- Cayenne pepper (to taste).
- 1 teaspoon chili powder.
- 2 eggs.
- 1 cup breadcrumbs (preferably seasoned).
- 1 cup uncooked brown rice.
- 1½ (15 ounces) can black beans, drained and rinsed.
- 1½ small onions, chopped (white or yellow).
- 1½ garlic cloves, minced.

Directions

- Mix the rice and 1 cup water in a small pot; bring to a boil and then turn down to medium heat and cook 20 minutes. Heat a little oil over medium heat in a saucepan and fry the onion and garlic for about 5 minutes.

- Add in the corn and spices and cook for another 5 minutes.
- Mash the drained beans with a fork in a medium bowl.
- Put the rice, corn, and onion, and mash it with a fork.
- Crack in the egg and mix it well.
- Add in the breadcrumbs.
- Make the patties by patting the desired amount of mixture into a flat round.
- Cook for about 2 minutes on each side.

Falafel with Tahini

10 Servings

Preparation Time: 1 hour 36 minutes

Ingredients

- 1½ teaspoons salt.
- 1 teaspoon chili powder
- 2½ teaspoons cumin.
- 2½ teaspoons baking powder.
- 1 cup all-purpose flour.
- Canola oil, for sautéing.
- Pita bread, for serving.
- 2½ cups roughly chopped white onion.
- 8 garlic cloves.
- 2½ cups cooked chickpeas, drained.
- 1½ cups lightly packed parsley leaves.
- 1½ cups lightly packed cilantro leaves.

Tahini Sauce:

- 2 cups plain yogurt (full fat or non-fat).
- 1 cup tahini (sesame paste).
- 2 ½ tablespoons fresh lemon juice.

Directions

- In the blender, add the onion and garlic cloves, and blend it. Transfer the mixture to a strainer to release the liquid, then let it set aside.

- In the bowl of a blender, add the chickpeas, parsley, cilantro, salt, chili powder, and blend it roughly.
- Put the onion mixture, baking powder in the blender and add flour in it and blend it; the mixture begins to form a small ball and is not sticky.
- Transfer the mixture to a bowl, wrap the plastic on it, and refrigerate it for about 1 hour.
- Now, prepare the tahini sauce by mixing the yogurt, tahini, and lemon juice. Spice it with salt and pepper, cover it and place it in the fridge.
- Now make small balls from the falafel mixture. And flatten them slightly, so they are the shape of patties.
- Put a large saucepan over medium heat and add a liberal amount of canola oil. Let the pan pre-heat for about 3 minutes, then add the falafel patties one by one, cook for 3 minutes from the side, then flip it and cook the other side until brown.
- Transfer the falafel patties to a paper towel-lined and season them with salt. Repeat this process until you have cooked all of the falafel.
- Place three or four falafel inside a halved, warmed pita and drizzle with the prepared tahini sauce.

Tangy Tomato Panini

6 Servings

Preparation Time: 1 hr and 20 minutes

Ingredients

- 2-3 cloves of garlic, crushed.
- 6 sandwich-sized chunks of ciabatta bread, cut in half horizontally.
- 1/2 cup pesto.
- 6 slices mozzarella cheese.
- 6 slices provolone cheese.
- 3 roma tomatoes, ends removed sliced 1/4" thick.
- Olive oil.
- Coarse kosher salt and freshly ground black pepper.

Directions

- Preheat the oven to 325ºF. Line the baking sheet with parchment paper and place the tomato slices in an even layer. Sprinkle with olive oil, salt, pepper, and crushed garlic. Bake it for about 65 minutes.
- Now heat a pan to medium-high. Spread the inside of all the bread with pesto, then place one slice of

mozzarella on the bottom piece of bread, add 4-6 tomato slices, and top with one slice of provolone. Replace the top piece of bread and grill sandwiches until crusty and melted for about 5 minutes.

Chicken Wraps

6 Servings

Preparation Time: 13 minutes

Ingredients

- 1½ cups your favorite marinara sauce.
- 1 cup finely chopped fresh basil.
- 4 flat-out flatbreads (we used light Italian herb).
- 1½ cups shredded, reduced-fat Italian cheese blend.
- Additional marinara sauce, warmed for dipping, if desired.
- 3½ cups roughly shredded, cooked boneless, skinless chicken breasts (see note).
- 2 teaspoons Italian seasoning (make sure yours is a salt-free blend).
- 1 teaspoon kosher salt.
- 1/8 teaspoon black pepper.

Directions

- Put shredded chicken in a medium bowl. Add in the Italian seasoning, salt, and black pepper, and mix it well.

- Add in the marinara sauce and basil to the chicken mixture, and stir to combine again.
- Put 1 flatbread on a work surface, and sprinkle 1/4 cup of cheese down the center, leaving a large border all around the cheese. Spread 1/4 of the chicken mixture
- Fold short ends of the flatbread inward toward the middle, and then fold the long sides of the flatbread inward toward the middle, making a closed wrap.
- Repeat the process with the remaining 3 flatbreads; divide the remaining cheese and the remaining chicken mixture evenly among them.
- Preheat a dry nonstick pan over medium heat. Add the wraps and cook on the first side until golden brown for about 1 1/2 - 2 minutes. Flip the wraps and cook the other side until golden, about another 1 1/2 minutes.
- Serve with an additional marinara sauce for dipping.

BRUNCH

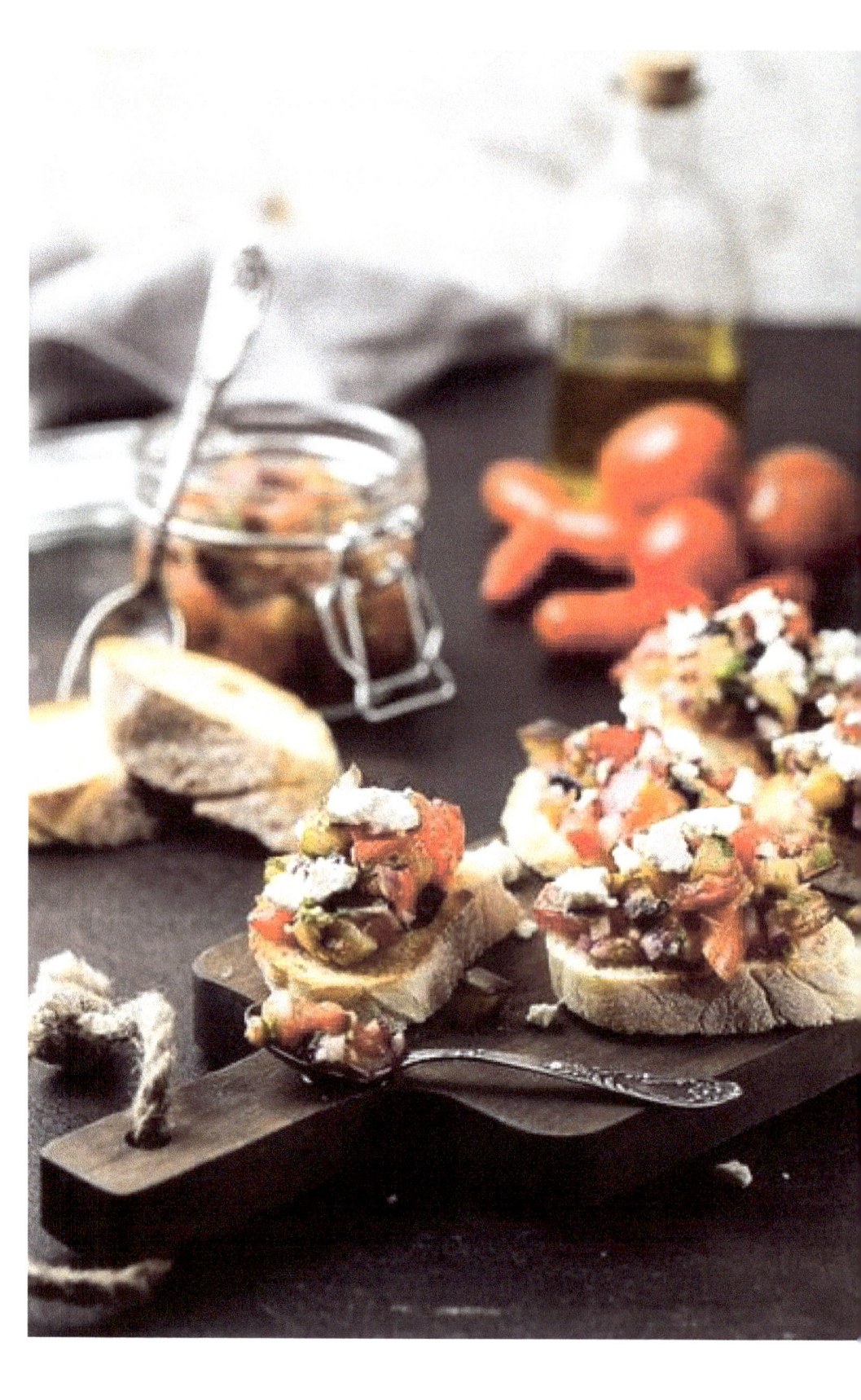

Lemon Artichokes

8 Servings

Preparation Time: 30 minutes

Ingredients

- 4 cups vegetable stock
- 2 tsps lemon zest, grated
- Pepper
- Salt
- 8 artichokes, trim and cut the top
- 0.5 cup fresh lemon juice

Directions

- This recipe Preparation begins with pouring the stock into the instant pot, then place the steamer rack in the pot.
- Place artichoke steam side down on steamer rack into the pot.
- Sprinkle lemon zest over artichokes. Season with pepper and salt.
- Pour lemon juice over artichokes.
- Seal pot with lid and cook on high for 20 minutes.

- Once done, allow to release pressure naturally for 5 minutes, then release remaining using quick release. Remove lid.
- Serve and enjoy.

Pepper Zucchinis

8 Servings

Preparation Time: 20 minutes

Ingredients

- 1 tsp cayenne
- 2 tbsps chili powder
- 0.5 cup vegetable stock
- Salt
- 8 zucchinis, cut into cubes
- 1 tsp red pepper flakes

Directions

- Add and mix all ingredients into the inner pot of instant pot and stir well.
- Seal pot with lid and cook on high for 10 minutes.
- Once done, allow to release pressure naturally for 10 minutes, then release remaining using quick release. Remove lid.
- Stir and serve.

Tasty Okra

8 Servings

Preparation Time: 20 minutes

Ingredients

- 2 tbsps paprika
- 2 cups can tomato, crushed
- Pepper
- Salt
- 4 cups okra, chopped
- 4 tbsps fresh dill, chopped

Directions

- Mix all ingredients into the inner pot of instant pot and stir well.
- Seal pot with lid and cook on high for 10 minutes.
- Once done, allow to release pressure naturally for 5 minutes, then release remaining using quick release. Remove lid.
- Stir well and serve.

Cauliflower with Dill

8 Servings

Preparation Time: 22 minutes

Ingredients

- 2 cups of can tomatoes, crushed
- 2 cups vegetable stock
- 2 tsps garlic, minced
- Pepper
- Salt
- 2 lbs cauliflower florets, chopped
- 2 tbsps fresh dill, chopped
- 0.5 tsp Italian seasoning
- 2 tbsps vinegar

Directions

- Mix all ingredients except dill into the instant pot and stir well.
- Seal pot with lid and cook on high for 12 minutes.

- Once done, allow to release pressure naturally for 10 minutes, then release remaining using quick release. Remove lid.
- Garnish with dill and serve.

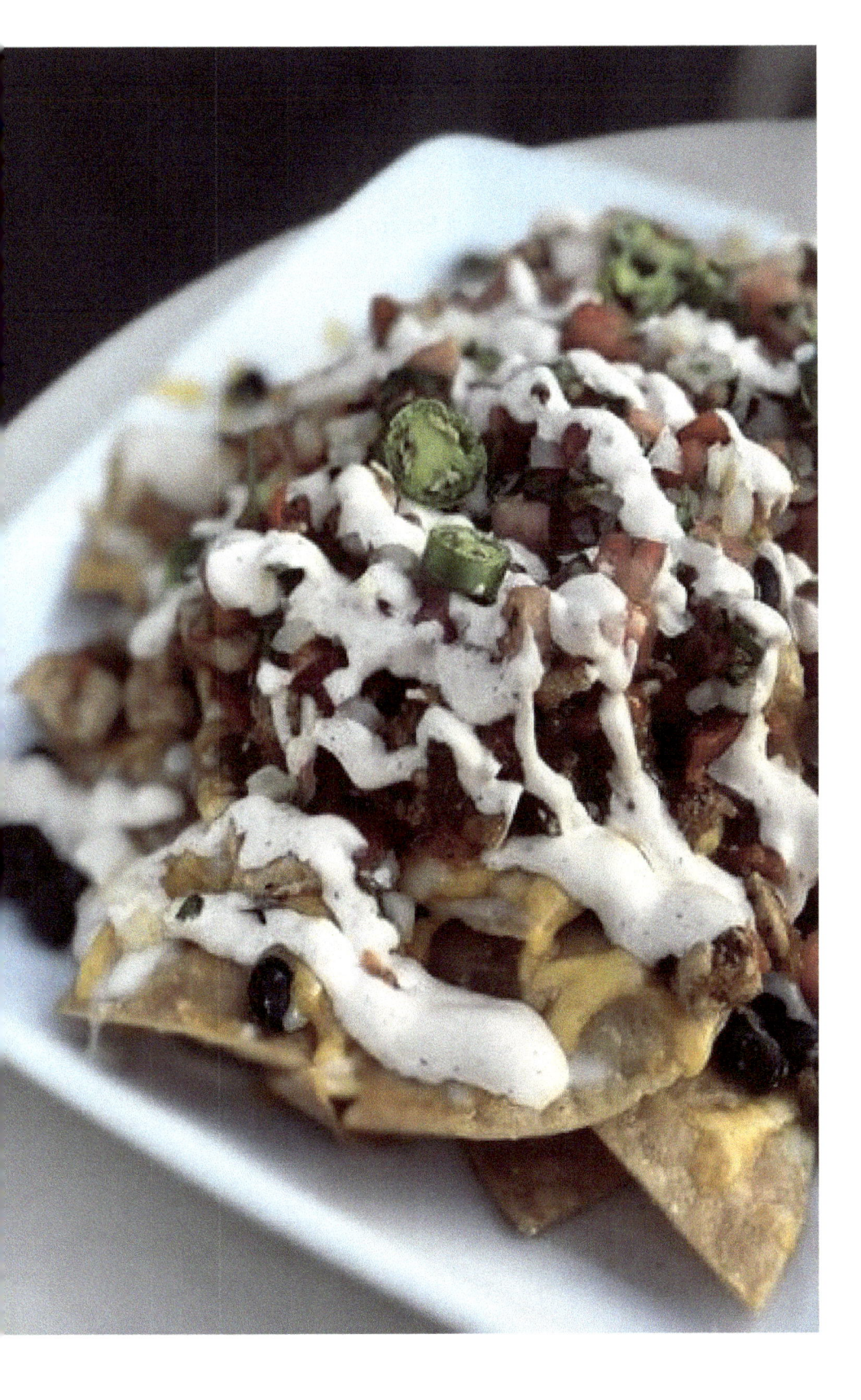

Eggplant with Parsnips

4 Servings

Preparation Time: 22 minutes

Ingredients
- 2 tsps of garlic, minced
- 2 eggplants, cut into chunks
- 0.5 tsp dried basil
- Pepper
- Salt
- 4 parsnips, sliced
- 2 cups can tomatoes, crushed
- 1 tsp ground cumin
- 2 tbsps paprika

Directions

- Mix all ingredients into the instant pot and stir well.
- Seal pot with lid and cook on high for 12 minutes.
- Once done, release pressure using quick release. Remove lid.
- Stir and serve.

Garlic Beans

4 Servings

Preparation Time: 15 minutes

Ingredients

- 2 tsps garlic, minced
- 2 tbsps olive oil
- Pepper
- Salt
- 2 lbs green beans, trimmed
- 1 cup vegetable stock

Directions

- Mix all ingredients into the instant pot and stir well.
- Seal pot with lid and cook on high for 5 minutes.
- Once done, release pressure using quick release. Remove lid.
- Stir and serve.

Olives with Eggplant

8 Servings

Preparation Time: 22 minutes

Ingredients

- 2 onions, chopped
- 2 tbsps olive oil
- 0.5 cup grape tomatoes
- Pepper
- Salt
- 8 cups eggplants, cut into cubes
- 1 cup vegetable stock
- 2 tsps chili powder
- 2 cups olives, pitted and sliced

Directions

- Take a pot and add oil into the inner pot of instant pot and set the pot on sauté mode.
- Add onion and sauté for 2 minutes.
- Add remaining ingredients and stir everything well.

- Seal pot with lid and cook on high for 12 minutes.
- Once done, allow to release pressure naturally for 10 minutes, then release remaining using quick release. Remove lid.
- Stir and serve.

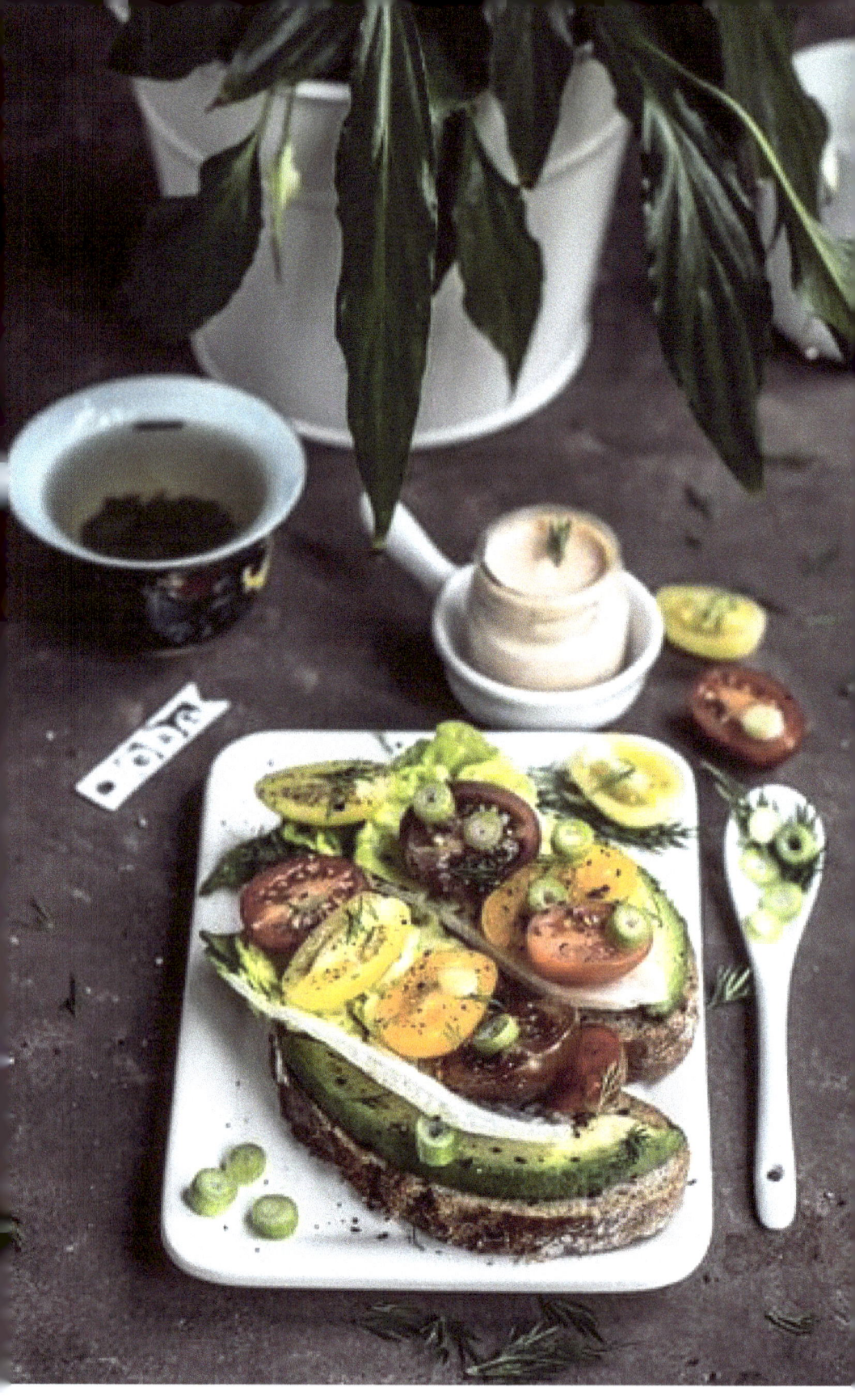

Broccoli & Vegan Carrots

12 Servings

Preparation Time: 15 minutes

Ingredients

- 2 tsps garlic, minced
- 2 tbsps olive oil
- 0.5 cup vegetable stock
- 0.5 tsp Italian seasoning
- Salt
- 8 cups broccoli florets
- 4 carrots, peeled and sliced
- 0.5 cup water
- 1 lemon juice

Directions

- Add oil into the inner pot of instant pot and set the pot on sauté mode.
- Add garlic and sauté for 30 seconds.
- Add carrots and broccoli and cook for 2 minutes.

- Add remaining ingredients and stir everything well.
- Seal pot with lid and cook on high for 3 minutes.
- Once done, release pressure using quick release. Remove lid.
- Stir well and serve

Seasonal Vegitable Ratatouille

12 Servings

Preparation Time: 20 minutes

Ingredients

- 2 bell peppers, diced
- 24 oz eggplant, diced
- 16 oz zucchini, diced
- 16 oz yellow squash, diced
- Pepper
- Salt
- 11 lbs potatoes, cut into cubes
- 1 cup fresh basil
- 56 oz fire-roasted tomatoes, chopped
- 2 onions, chopped
- 8 mushrooms, sliced

Directions

- Mix all ingredients except basil into the instant pot and stir well.
- Seal pot with lid and cook on high for 10 minutes.

- Once done, release pressure using quick release. Remove lid.
- Add basil and stir well and serve.

Coconut Clam Chowder

12 Servings

Preparation Time: 17 minutes

Ingredients

- 2 cups fish broth
- 2 bay leaves
- 4 cups of coconut milk
- Salt
- 12 oz clams, chopped
- 2 cups heavy cream
- 0.5 onion, sliced
- 2 cups celery, chopped
- 2 lbs cauliflower, chopped

Directions

- Mix all ingredients except clams and heavy cream and stir well.
- Seal pot with lid and cook on high for 5 minutes.
- Once done, release pressure using quick release. Remove lid.

- Add heavy cream and clams and stir well and cook on sauté mode for 2 minutes.
- Stir well and serve.

DINNER

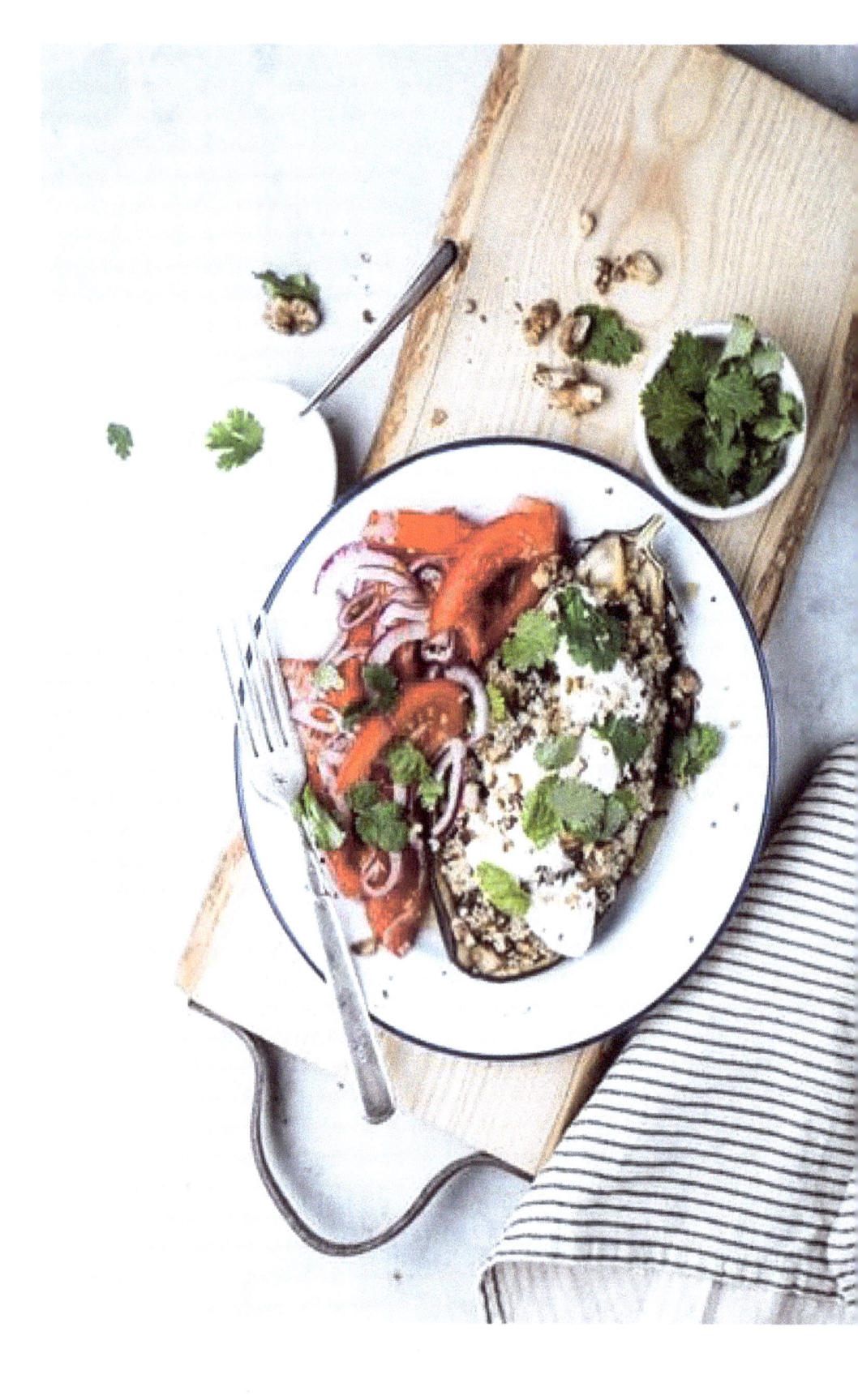

Vegetable Stew

6 Servings

Preparation Time: 32 minutes

Ingredients

- 1½ heads of cauliflower, cut into florets
- 3 cups green beans, halved
- 3 tbsps olive oil
- 1½ garlic cloves, minced
- 2 cups crème fraîch
- 1½ onions, chopped
- 3 carrots, chopped
- 1½ cups of water
- Salt and black pepper to taste

Directions

- Heat the olive oil in a saucepan over medium heat and fry the garlic and onion to be fragrant for about 3 minutes.
- Add in carrots, cauliflower, and green beans, salt, and pepper, add the water, stir again, now cook the vegetables on low heat for about 25 minutes to be softened.
- Stir in the heavy cream to be combined, turn the heat off, and adjust the taste with salt and pepper and then serve.

Classical Spinach & Feta Lasagna

6 Servings

Preparation Time: 50 minutes

Ingredients

- 30 oz canned tomato sauce
- 10 oz baby spinach
- 3 pounds zucchinis, sliced
- Salt and black pepper to taste
- 3 cups feta cheese, crumbled
- 3 cups mozzarella cheese, shredded

Directions

- With the cooking spray grease the baking dish.
- Evenly combine the feta, mozzarella, salt, and pepper, and spread ¼ cup of the mixture in the bottom of the baking dish.
- Layer the ⅓ of zucchini slices on the top, spread 1 cup of tomato sauce over, and scatter a ⅓ of the spinach on top.
- Repeat this layering process, making sure to layer with the last ¼ cup of cheese mixture finally.

- Grease one end of foil with cooking spray and cover the baking dish with the foil.
- Bake it in the oven for 35 minutes at 370ºF; after that, remove foil, and bake further for about 5 to 10 minutes until the cheese has a nice golden brown color.
- Transfer it to the dish, let it set for 5 minutes, make slices of the lasagna, and serve warm.

Sage Flan and Green Beans

6 Servings

Preparation Time: 65 minutes

Ingredients

- 3 tbsps butter, melted
- 1½ tbsps butter, softened
- 1½ cups green beans, ends removed
- 1 cup whipping cream
- 3 tbsps fresh sage, chopped
- Salt and black pepper to taste
- 1½ cups of milk
- 3 eggs + 3 egg yolks, beaten in a bowl
- A small pinch of nutmeg
- 3 tbsps parmesan cheese, grated
- 6 cups of water

Directions

- Put 1 cup of the water and some salt in a pot, add the green beans, then allow it to boil over medium heat for about 6 minutes.
- Drain the green beans, and cut them into small pieces.

- Add the chopped green beans, whipping cream, milk, sage, salt, nutmeg, black pepper, and Parmesan cheese in the blender.
- Blend the ingredients at high speed until smooth.
- Put the mixture into a bowl and whisk the eggs into it.
- Preheat the oven to 350ºF.
- Brush the baking dish with softened butter and spread the green bean mixture in it.
- Spread the melted butter over each mixture.
- Pour the remaining water into a baking dish; put the baking dish in the oven.
- Bake for about 45 minutes until their middle parts are no longer watery.
- Remove the baking dish and let it cool.

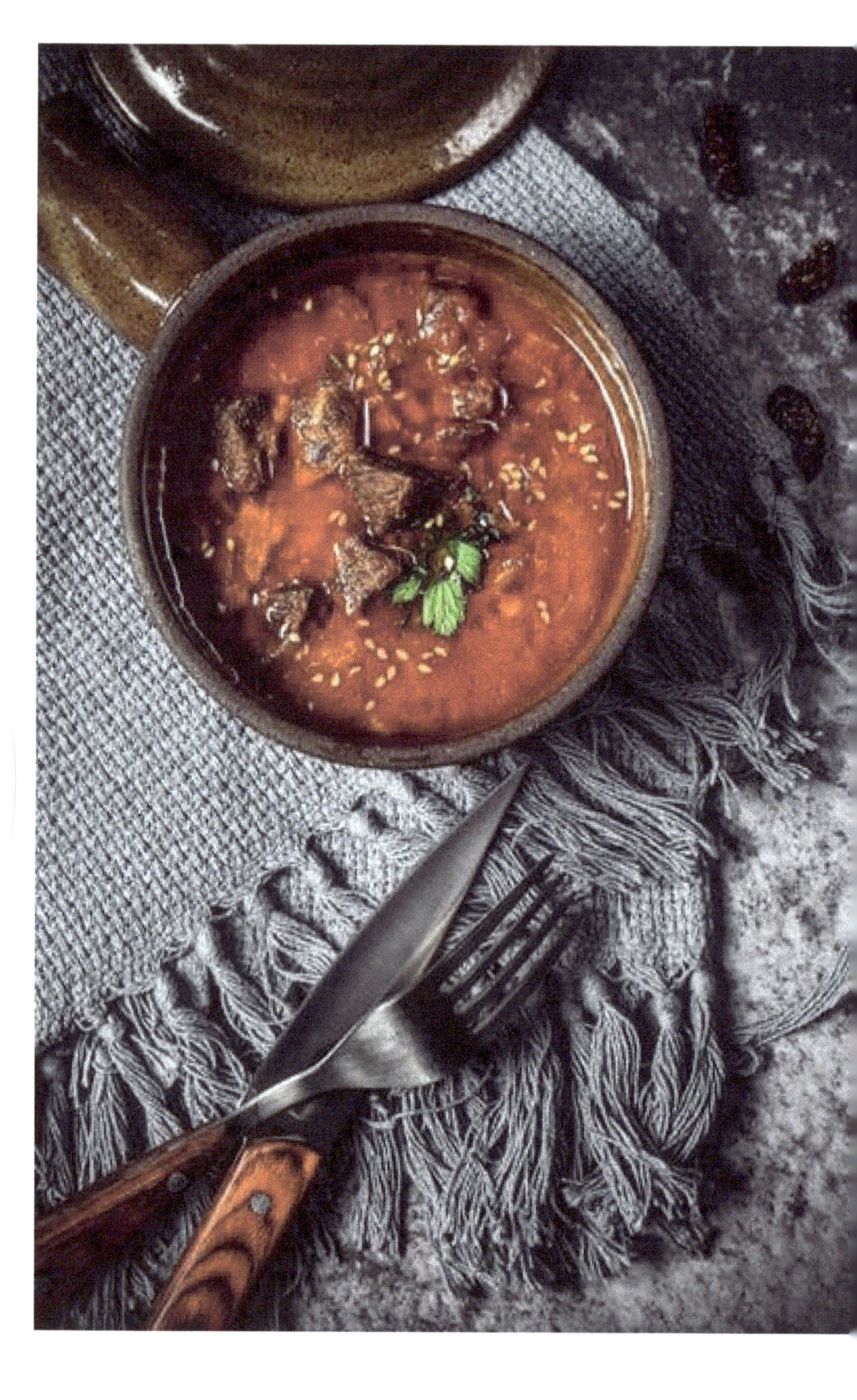

Grilled Cauliflower Steaks & Steamed Asparagus

6 Servings

Preparation Time: 20 minutes

Ingredients

- Juice of 1½ lemons
- 1½ cups of water
- Dried parsley to garnish
- 6 tbsps olive oil
- 3 heads cauliflower, sliced into 'steaks'
- 3 tsps sugar
- Salt and black pepper to taste
- 1½ red onions, sliced
- 1 cup chili sauce
- 1½ pounds asparagus, trimmed

Directions

- Preheat the grill.
- Mix the olive oil, chili sauce, and sugar in a bowl. Brush the cauliflower with the mixture.

- Put them on the grill, and cook for about 6 minutes. Flip the cauliflower on it, grill for another 6 minutes.
- Boil the water over high heat, put the asparagus in a strainer, and let it set.
- Cook for about 6 minutes. Transfer it to a bowl and shower with lemon juice.
- Transfer the grilled caulis on a plate; sprinkle some salt, black pepper, red onion, and parsley.
- Serve with the steamed asparagus.

Green Bell Pepper & Mushroom Stew

6 Servings

Preparation Time: 25 minutes

Ingredients

- 1½ tsps paprika
- 3 tomatoes, chopped
- 1½ tbsps flaxseed meal
- 3 tbsps olive oil
- 1½ onions, chopped
- 3 carrots, chopped
- 10 oz wild mushrooms, sliced
- 3 tbsps dry white wine
- 3 garlic cloves, pressed
- 1 stalk celery, chopped
- 1½ thyme sprig, chopped
- 5 cups vegetable stock
- 1 tsp chili pepper

Directions

- Heat the oil in a stockpot over medium heat.
- Stir in the onion and cook until tender.

- Put in the carrots, celery, and garlic and fry until soft for 4 more minutes.
- Add in the mushrooms; cook the mixture until the liquid is lost; then let the vegetables set aside.
- Pour in wine to deglaze the stockpot's bottom. Put in the thyme.
- Add in tomatoes, vegetable stock, paprika, and chili pepper; add in the vegetables and allow boiling.
- On low heat, allow the mixture to simmer for about 15 minutes.
- Add in the flaxseed meal to thicken the stew.
- Serve into the individual bowls.

Traditional Spanish Pisto

8 Servings

Preparation Time: 47 minutes

Ingredients

- 5 sprigs thyme
- 1½ tbsps balsamic vinegar
- 5 tbsps olive oil
- 8 eggs
- 4 zucchinis, chopped
- 2½ eggplants, chopped
- 2½ red bell peppers, cut in chunks
- 1½ yellow bell peppers, cut in chunks
- 4 cloves of garlic, sliced
- 2½ onions, diced
- Zest of ½ lemon
- 32 oz canned tomatoes

Directions

- Heat 1 tbsp of olive oil in a pan and fry the eggs; transfer it on a platter, then cover with aluminum foil to keep warm and let it set aside.
- In a large pan, warm the remaining olive oil and fry the eggplants, zucchinis, and bell peppers over

medium heat for about 5 minutes. After fry place the veggies into a large bowl.

- Add the garlic, onions, and thyme leaves in the same pan and cook for about 5 minutes.
- Returned the cooked veggies to the pan along with the canned tomatoes, balsamic vinegar, chopped basil, salt, and pepper to taste.
- Cook the ingredients on low heat for about 30 minutes, and then cover it with the lid.
- Now open the lid and add in the remaining basil leaves, lemon zest, and adjust the seasoning.
- Turn the heat off. Plate the ratatouille and serve with fried eggs.

Greek Salad with Dill Dressing

6 Servings

Preparation Time: 3 hrs 15 minutes

Ingredients

For the Dressing

- Salt and black pepper, to taste
- 1 tsp dill, minced
- 3 tbsps of milk
- 3 tbsps green onions, chopped
- 3 cups water
- 1½ garlic cloves, minced
- 1 lemon, freshly squeezed

For the salad

- 3 tbsps kalamata olives, pitted
- 6 oz feta cheese, crumbled
- 1½ head lettuce, torn
- 4 tomatoes, diced
- 4 cucumbers, sliced

Directions

- Mix the lettuce, olives, red onion, tomato, cucumber, and feta in a large bowl.

- Add all dressing ingredients into a food processor and blend it well.
- Add the dressing to the salad and shake.

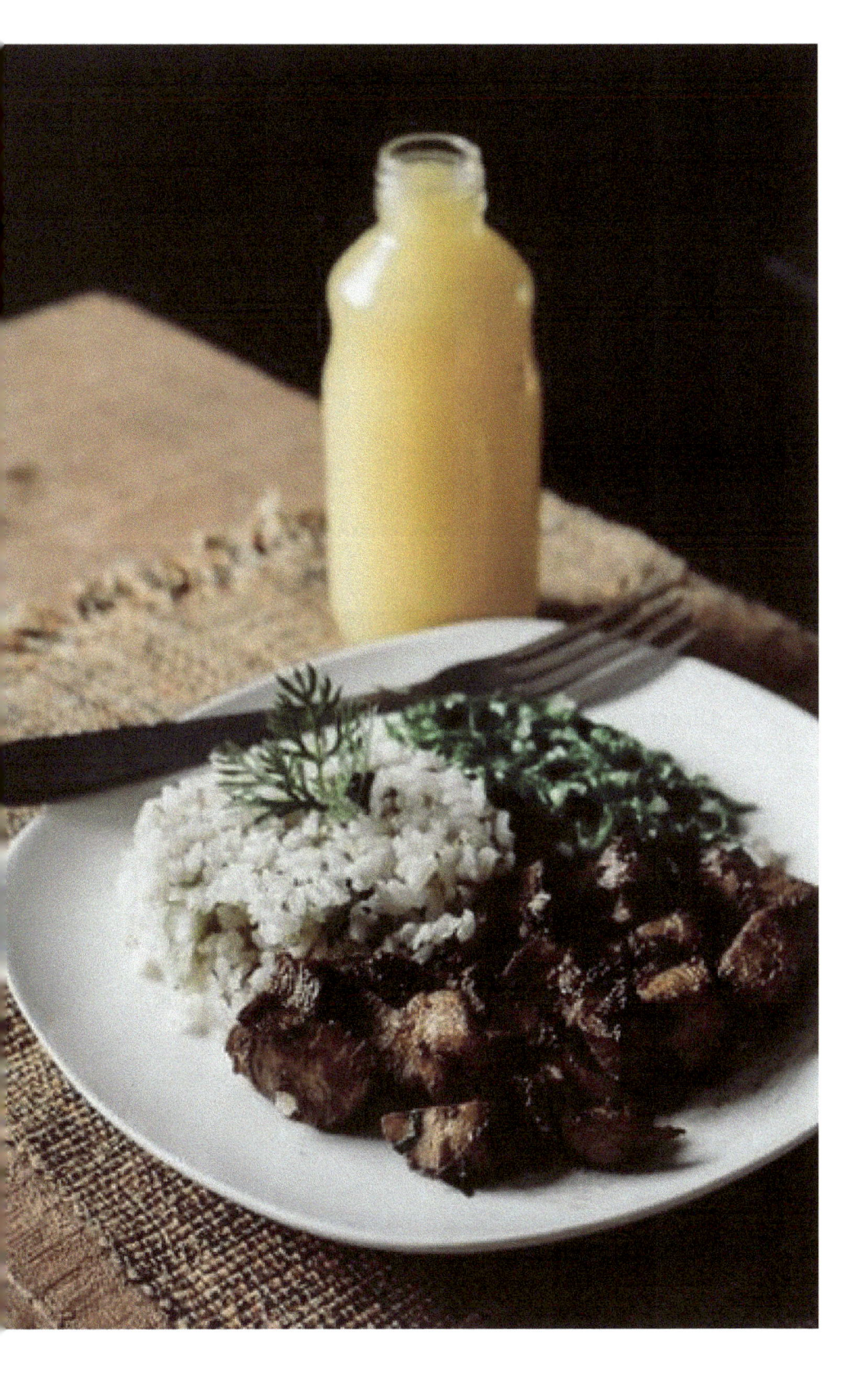

Zucchini Spaghetti and Avocado & Capers

6 Servings

Preparation Time: 15 minutes

Ingredients

- 3 avocados, sliced
- 1 cup capers
- 1 cup sun-dried tomatoes, chopped
- 2½ tbsps olive oil
- 1½ pounds zucchinis, julienned
- 1 cup pesto

Directions

- Warm half of the olive oil in a pan over medium heat.
- Stir the zucchinis and fry for about 4 minutes. Transfer it to the plate.
- Add in pesto, salt, tomatoes, and capers.
- Top with avocado slices.

Vegan Minestrone

7 Servings

Preparation Time: 25 minutes

Ingredients

- 7 cups vegetable broth
- 1½ cups baby spinach
- Salt and black pepper to taste
- 3 tbsps olive oil
- 1½ small onions, chopped
- 1½ garlic cloves, minced
- 3 heads broccoli, cut in florets
- 3 stalks celery, chopped

Directions

- Fry the onion and garlic in a saucepan over medium heat for about 3 minutes until softened.
- Stir in the broccoli and celery, and cook for about 4 minutes until slightly tender.
- Pour in the broth, boil it, then reduce the heat to medium-low and simmer covered for about 5 minutes.

- Add in the spinach to wilt, adjust the spices, and cook for about 4 minutes.
- Serve the soup into the bowls.

Kale & Cauliflower Cheese Waffles

5 Servings

Preparation Time: 45 minutes

Ingredients

- 1 cauliflower head
- 1½ tsps garlic powder
- 1½ tbsps sesame seeds
- 3 tsps rosemary, chopped
- 3 spring onions, chopped
- 1½ tbsps olive oil
- 3 eggs
- 1 cup Parmesan cheese, shredded
- 10 oz kale, chopped
- 1½ cups mozzarella cheese, shredded

Directions

- Put the chopped cauliflower in the food processor and blend until rice is formed.
- Add the kale, spring onions, and rosemary into the food processor. Blend until smooth. Transfer it to the bowl. Add in the rest of the ingredients and mix to combine.

- Warm the waffle iron and evenly spread in ¼ of the mixture.
- Cook until golden for about 3 minutes.
- Repeat the process with the remaining batter.

DESSERT

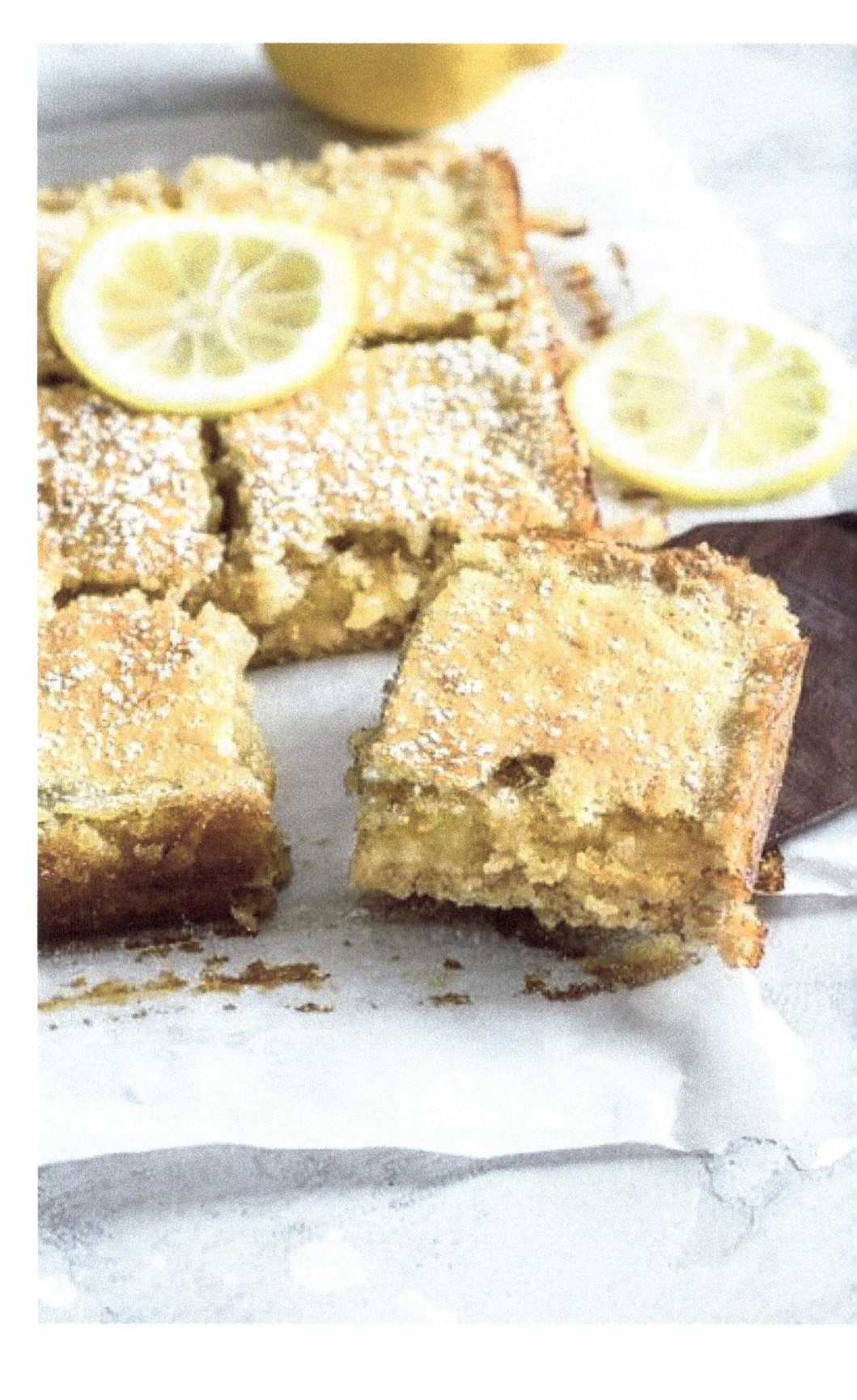

Almond Rice

4 Servings

Preparation Time: 20 minutes

Ingredients

- 1 cup white rice
- 2 cups almond milk
- 1 cup almonds, chopped.
- Half cup stevia
- 1 tablespoon cinnamon powder
- Half cup pomegranate seeds.

Directions:

- In a pot, mix the rice with the milk and stevia, bring to a simmer, and cook for 20 minutes, mixing often.
- Add the rest of the ingredients, mix, divide into bowls and serve.

Frozen Strawberry Yogurt

16 Servings

Preparation Time: 15 minutes

Ingredients

- 3 cups Greek yogurt, plain, low-fat (2%)
- 2 tsps vanilla
- 1/8 tsp. salt
- 1/4 cup freshly squeezed lemon juice
- 1 cup sugar
- 1 cup strawberries, sliced.

Directions:

- In a medium-sized bowl, except for the strawberries, combine the rest of the ingredients.
- Whisking until the mixture is smooth.
- Transfer the yogurt into a 1 Half or 2-quart ice cream maker and freeze according to the manufacturer's direction, adding the strawberry slices for the last minute.
- Transfer into an airtight container and freeze for about 2-4 hours.
- Before serving, let stand for 15 minutes at room temperature.

Almond Peaches

4 Servings

Preparation Time: 10 minutes

Ingredients

- 1/3 cup almonds, toasted.
- 1/3 cup pistachios, toasted.
- 1 tsp. mint, chopped.
- Half cup coconut water
- 1 tsp. lemon zest, grated.
- 4 peaches, halved.
- 2 tbsps stevia

Directions:

- In a pan, combine the peaches with the stevia and the rest of the ingredients.
- Simmer over medium heat for 10 minutes, divide into bowls and serve cold.

Raisin Baked Apples

6 Servings

Preparation Time: 4 minutes

Ingredients

- 6 apples cored and cut into wedges.
- 1 cup red wine
- 1/4 cup pecans, chopped.
- 1/4 cup raisins
- 1/4 tsp nutmeg
- 1 tsp cinnamon
- 1/3 cup honey

Directions:

- Add all ingredients into the instant pot and mix well.
- Seal pot with lid and cook on high for 4 minutes.
- Once done, allow to release pressure naturally for 10 minutes, then release remaining using quick release.
- Remove lid.
- Mix well and serve.

Walnuts Sweet Cake

4 Servings

Preparation Time: 40 minutes

Ingredients
- Half pound walnuts, minced.
- Zest of 1 orange, grated.
- 1 and ¼ cups stevia
- Eggs, whisked.
- 1 tsp. almond extract
- 1 and half cup almond flour
- 1 tsp. baking soda

Directions:

- In a bowl, combine the walnuts with the orange zest and the other ingredients.
- Whisk well and transfer into a cake pan lined with parchment paper.
- Introduce in the oven at 350 degrees F, bake for 40 minutes, cool down, slice, and serve.

Tasty Cookies

6 Servings

Preparation Time: 30 minutes

Ingredients

- 1 egg, beaten.
- 1 tsp. vanilla extract
- Half tsp ground cinnamon
- 1 tsp ground turmeric
- 1 tablespoon butter, softened.
- 1 cup wheat flour
- 1 tsp baking powder
- 4 tbsps pumpkin puree
- 1 tablespoon Erythritol

Directions:

- Put all ingredients in the mixing bowl and knead the soft and non-sticky dough.
- After this, line the baking tray with baking paper.
- Make 6 balls from the dough and press them gently with the help of the spoon.
- Arrange the dough balls in the tray.
- Bake the cookies for 30 minutes at 355F.
- Chill the cooked cookies well and store them in the glass jar.

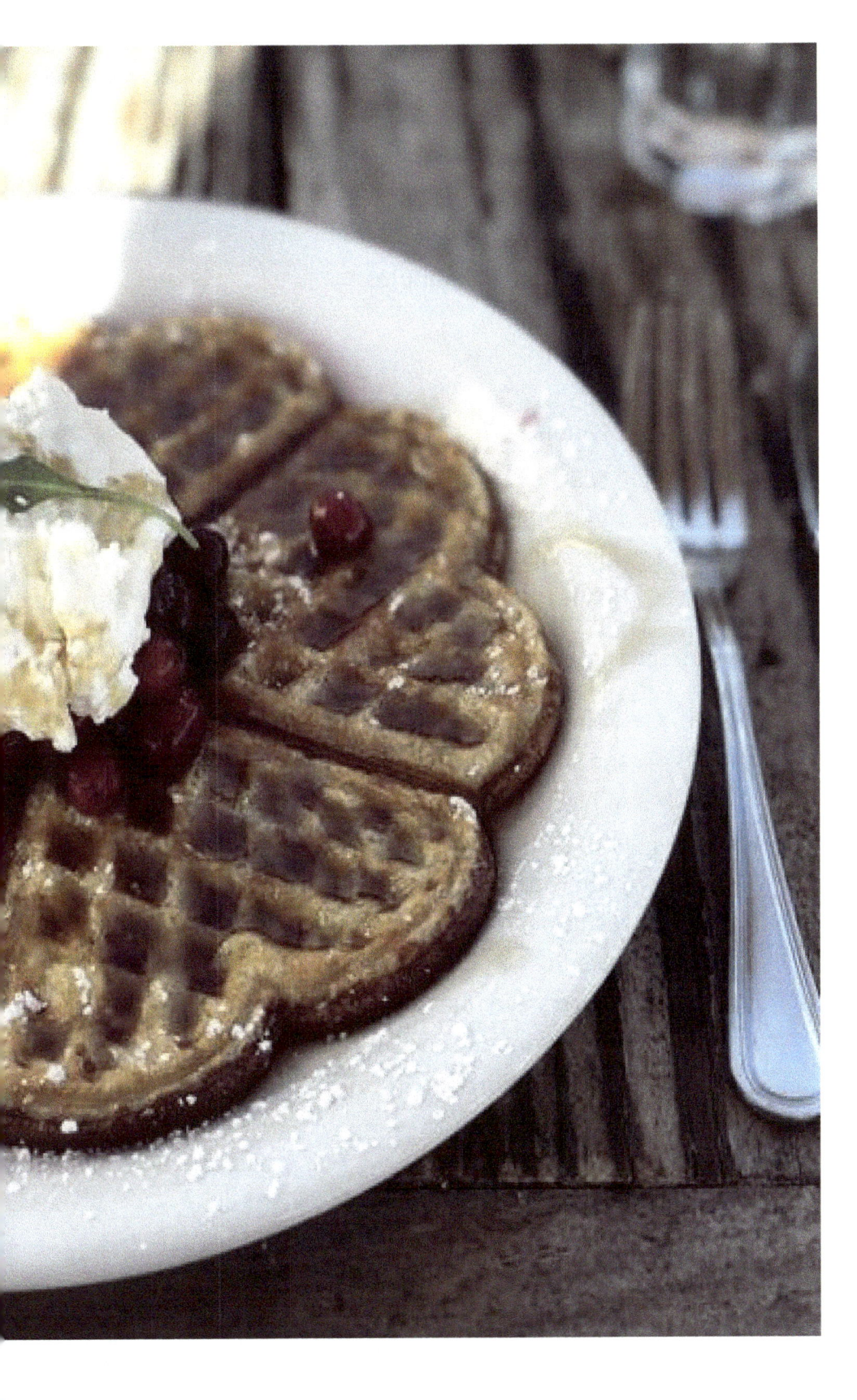

Cinnamon Cakes

8 Servings

Preparation Time: 40 minutes

Ingredients

- 1 lemon
- 4 eggs
- 1 tsp cinnamon
- ¼ lb. sugar
- Half lb. ground almonds

Directions:

- Preheat oven to 350oF. Then grease a cake pan and set it aside.
- At high speed, beat for three minutes the sugar and eggs or until the volume is doubled.
- Then with a spatula, gently fold in the lemon zest, cinnamon, and almond flour until well mixed.
- Then transfer batter on prepared pan and bake for forty minutes or until golden brown.
- Let cool before serving.

Yummy Yogurt Cake

1 Serving

Preparation Time: 55 minutes

Ingredients

- 1 cup plain Greek yogurt
- 1 cup sugar
- 2 large eggs
- 1 tablespoon vanilla extract
- 4 tablespoons fresh lemon juice
- 1 tablespoon lemon zest
- Half cup vegetable or light olive oil
- 1 three quarters cups all-purpose flour
- 2 tsps. baking powder
- Half tsp salt.
- 1 cup of confectioners' sugar

Directions:

- Preheat the oven to 350ºF. Lightly coat a 9-inch-round cake pan with cooking spray, and dust the pan using about 2 tbsps of all-purpose flour.
- In a large bowl, using an electric mixer on medium speed, Keep blending Greek yogurt, sugar, eggs, vanilla extract, 2 tbsp. lemon juice,

lemon zest, and vegetable oil for about 2 minutes.
- Add all-purpose flour, baking powder, and salt, and Keep blending for 2 more minutes.
- Transfer batter into the prepared cake pan and bake for 55 minutes or until a toothpick inserted in the center of the cake comes out clean.
- Cool cake completely.
- In a small bowl, whisk together confectioners' sugar and the remaining 2 tbsps of lemon juice to make a glaze.
- When cake is cool, transfer glaze over the top, cut, and serve.

Apple Sauce with Chunks

16 Servings

Preparation Time: 12 minutes

Ingredients

- 4 apples, peeled, cored, and diced.
- 1 tsp vanilla
- 4 pears, diced.
- 2 tbsps cinnamon
- 1/4 cup maple syrup
- Three quarters cup water

Directions:

- Add all ingredients into the instant pot and mix well.
- Seal pot with lid and cook on high for 12 minutes.
- Once done, allow to release pressure naturally for 10 minutes, then release remaining using quick release.
- Remove lid.
- Serve and enjoy.

Olives Cake

1 Serving

Preparation Time: 45 minutes

Ingredients

- 2 large eggs
- Three quarters cup sugar
- Half cup light olive oil
- 1 cup plain Greek yogurt
- 3 tablespoons fresh orange juice
- 2 tablespoons orange zest
- 1 three-quarters cups all-purpose flour
- Half tsp. salt.
- 2 tsps. baking powder
- Half tsp. baking soda
- Three-quarters cup dried cranberries
- 2 tablespoons of confectioners' sugar

Directions:

- Preheat the oven to 350ºF. Lightly coat a 9-inch-round cake pan or Bundt pan with cooking spray, and dust with about 2 tbsps of all purpose flour.

- In a large bowl, and using an electric mixer on medium speed, Keep blending eggs and sugar for 2 minutes.
- Keep blending in light olive oil, Greek yogurt, orange juice, and orange zest for 2 more minutes.
- Add all-purpose flour, salt, baking powder, and baking soda, and Keep blending for 1 more minute.
- Using a spatula or wooden spoon, fold cranberries into batter.
- Transfer batter into the prepared pan and bake for 45 minutes or until a toothpick inserted in the center of the cake comes out clean.
- Cool cake completely.
- Dust top of the cake with confectioners' sugar, cut, and serve.

SALADS AND SOUPS

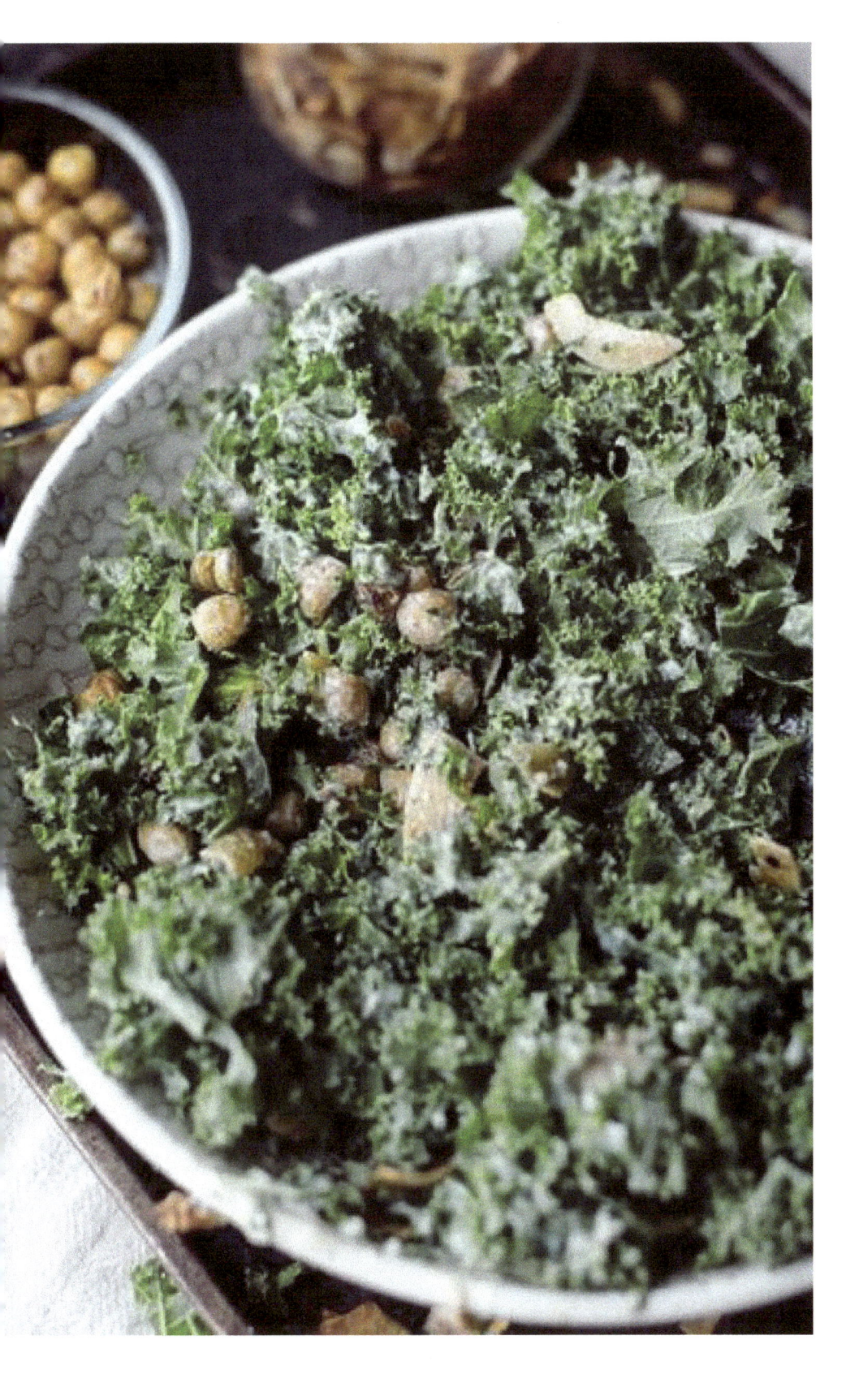

Pinto Bean Salad

8 Servings

Preparation Time: 30 minutes

Ingredients

- 3½ tablespoons lemon juice.
- 1½ tablespoons ground dried Aleppo pepper.
- 8 ounces cherry tomatoes halved.
- 1½ cups (6 ounces) orchard choice or sun-maid California figs stemmed and halved.
- 2 red onions thinly sliced.
- 2 cups of fresh parsley leaves.
- 2½ large hard-cooked eggs quartered.
- 1½ tablespoons toasted sesame seeds.
- 1 cup extra virgin-olive oil.
- 3½ garlic cloves lightly crushed and peeled.
- 2 ½ (15 ounces) cans pinto beans rinsed.
- Salt and pepper.
- 1/4 cup tahini.

Directions

- Add 1 tablespoon oil and garlic in a medium saucepan over medium heat, stir it often, until garlic turns golden but not brown, about 3

minutes. Add in the beans, 2 cups water, and 1 teaspoon salt and bring to simmer. Remove from heat, cover, and let sit for about 20 minutes.
- Strain the beans and discard garlic. Mix the remaining 3 tablespoons of oil, tahini, lemon juice, Aleppo pepper, 1 tablespoon water, and 1/4 teaspoon salt in a large bowl.
- Add in beans, tomatoes, figs, onion, and parsley, and gently mix it. Spice with salt and pepper. Transfer it to a serving platter and put eggs on top. Sprinkle with sesame seeds and extra Aleppo pepper and serve.

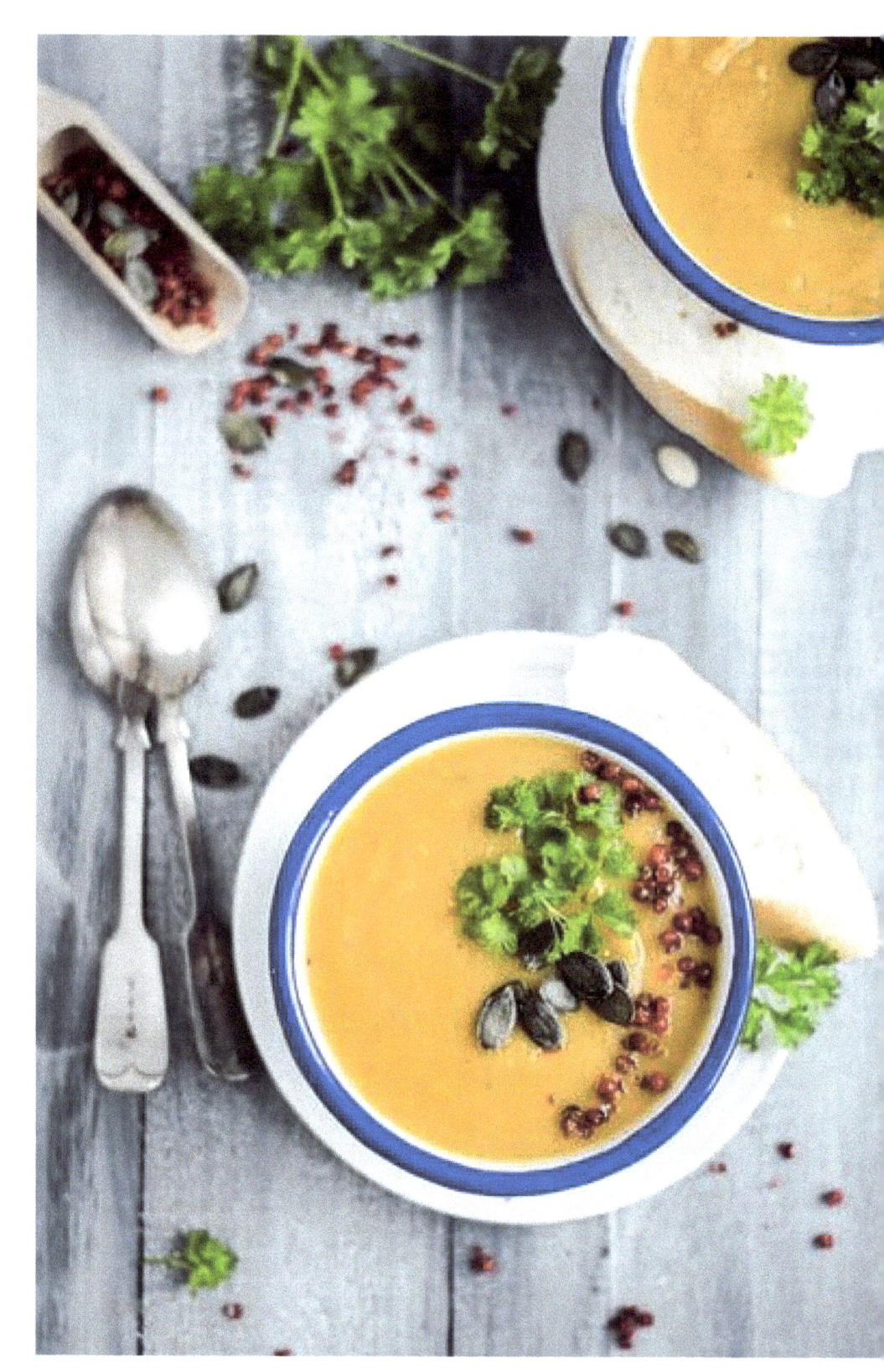

Chicken Salad Pitas

6 Servings

Preparation Time: 15 minutes

Ingredients

- 1 teaspoon red pepper, crushed
- 1 cup fresh cilantro, chopped
- 1 teaspoon ground cumin
- 1 cup red onion, diced
- 1 cup (about 20 small) green olives, chopped, pitted
- 1½ cups Greek yogurt, plain, whole-milk
- 1½ cups (about 1 large) red bell pepper, chopped
- 8 pieces (6-inch) whole-wheat pitas, cut into halves
- 8 slices (1/8-inch-thick) tomato, cut into halves
- 1½ cans (15-ounce) chickpeas (garbanzo beans), no-salt-added, rinsed, drained
- 4 cups chicken, cooked, chopped
- 2½ tablespoons lemon juice
- 14 Bibb lettuce leaves

Directions

- In a small bowl, combine the yogurt, lemon juice, cumin, and red pepper; set aside.
- In a large mixing bowl, combine the chicken, red bell pepper, olives, red onion, cilantro, and chickpeas. Add the yogurt mixture into the chicken mixture; gently toss to coat.
- Line each pita half with 1 lettuce leaf and then with 1 tomato slice. Fill each pita half with 1/2 cup of the chicken mixture.

Mulligatawny Soup

20 Servings

Preparation time: 30 minutes

Ingredients

- 20 cups chicken broth
- 10 cups chicken, chopped and cooked
- 0.5 cup apple cider
- 0.5 cup sour cream
- 0.5 cup fresh parsley, chopped
- 4 tablespoons butter
- Salt and black pepper, to taste
- 6 tablespoons curry powder
- 6 cups celery root, diced
- 4 tablespoons Swerve

Directions

- Mix the broth, butter, chicken, curry powder, celery root, and apple cider in a large soup pot.
- Bring to a boil and simmer for about 30 minutes.
- Stir in Swerve, sour cream, fresh parsley, salt, and black pepper.
- Dish out and serve hot.

Ranch Chicken Soup

8 Servings

Preparation time: 40 minutes

Ingredients

- 2 cups heavy whipping cream
- 8 cups chicken, cooked and shredded
- 8 tablespoons ranch dressing
- 0.5 cup yellow onions, chopped
- 16 oz cream cheese
- 16 cups chicken broth
- 14 hearty bacon slices, crumbled
- 4 tablespoons parsley
- 4 celery stalks, chopped
- 12 tablespoons butter

Directions

- Heat butter in a pan and add chicken.
- Cook for about 5 minutes and add 1½ cups water.
- Cover and cook for about 10 minutes.

- Now put the chicken and the rest of the ingredients into the saucepan except parsley and cook for about 10 minutes.
- Top with parsley and serve hot.

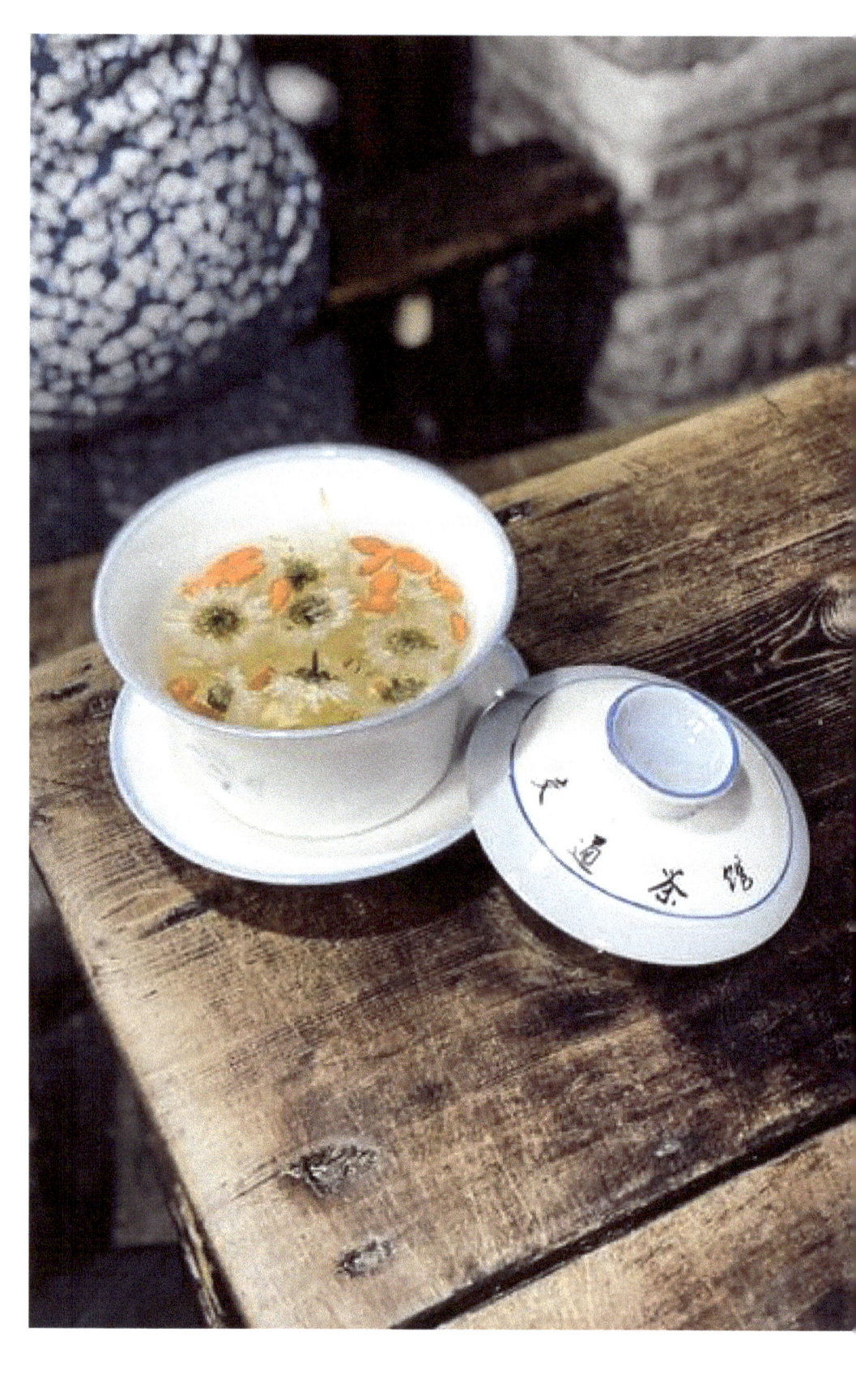

Classical Chicken Soup

12 Servings

Preparation time: 1 hour 45 minutes

Ingredients

- 0.6 large red onion
- 2 large carrots
- 6 garlic cloves
- 4 thyme sprigs
- 4 rosemary sprigs
- Salt and black pepper, to taste
- 6 pounds chicken
- 8 quarts water
- 8 stalks celery

Directions

- Put water and chicken in the stock pot on medium-high heat.
- Bring to a boil and allow it to simmer for about 10 minutes.
- Add onion, garlic, celery, salt, and pepper and simmer on medium-low heat for 30 minutes.

- Add thyme and carrots and simmer on low for another 30 minutes.
- Dish out the chicken and shred the pieces, removing the bones.
- Return the chicken pieces to the pot and add rosemary sprigs.
- Simmer for about 20 minutes at low heat and dish out to serve.

Soothing Chicken Noodle Soup

12 Servings

Preparation time: 30 minutes

Ingredients

- 6 cups chicken, shredded
- 6 eggs, lightly beaten
- 2 green onions, for garnish
- 4 tablespoons coconut oil
- 2 carrots, peeled and thinly sliced
- 4 teaspoons dried thyme
- 10 quarts homemade bone broth
- 0.5 cup fresh parsley, minced
- Salt and black pepper, to taste
- 2 onions, minced
- 2 rib celeries, sliced

Directions

- Now heat coconut oil over medium-high heat in a large pot and add onions, carrots, and celery.

- Cook for about 4 minutes and stir in the bone broth, thyme, and chicken.
- Simmer for about 15 minutes and stir in parsley.
- Pour beaten eggs into the soup in a slow, steady stream.
- Remove soup from heat and let it stand for about 2 minutes.
- Season with salt and black pepper and dish out to serve.

Cabbage and Chicken Soup

16 Servings

Preparation time: 35 minutes

Ingredients
- 16 cups chicken broth
- 2 medium carrots
- 4 cups green cabbage, sliced into strips
- 4 teaspoons dried parsley
- 0.5 teaspoon black pepper
- 10 rotisserie chickens, shredded
- 4 celery stalks
- 4 garlic cloves, minced
- 8 oz butter
- 12 oz. mushrooms, sliced
- 4 tablespoons onions, dried and minced
- 2 teaspoons of salt

Directions

- In a large pot and melt the butter in it and add celery, mushrooms, onions and garlic into the pot.

- Cook for about 4 minutes and add broth, parsley, carrot, salt, and black pepper.
- Simmer for about 10 minutes and add cooked chicken and cabbage.
- Simmer for an additional 12 minutes until the cabbage is tender.
- Dish out and serve hot.

Enchilada Soup

10 Servings

Preparation time: 20 minutes

Ingredients

- 2 cups cheddar cheese, shredded
- 4 cups cooked chicken, shredded
- 4 cups chicken stock
- 8 oz. cream cheese, softened
- 1 cup salsa Verde

Directions

- Take and put salsa Verde, cheddar cheese, cream cheese, and chicken stock in an immersion blender and blend until smooth.
- Pour this mixture into a medium saucepan and cook for about 5 minutes on medium heat.
- Add the shredded chicken and cook for about 5 minutes.
- Garnish with additional shredded cheddar and serve hot.

BBQ Chicken Pizza Soup

12 Servings

Preparation time: 1 hour 30 minutes

Ingredients

- 8 cups green beans
- 1.5 cup BBQ Sauce
- 10 cups mozzarella cheese, shredded
- 0.5 cup ghee
- 4 quarts water
- 4 quarts chicken stock
- Salt and black pepper, to taste
- Fresh cilantro, for garnishing
- 12 chicken legs
- 2 medium red onions, diced
- 8 garlic cloves
- 2 large tomatoes, unsweetened

Directions

- Keep chicken, water, and salt in a large pot and bring to a boil.

- Reduce the heat to medium-low and cook for about 75 minutes.
- Shred the meat off the bones using a fork and keep aside.
- Put ghee, red onions, and garlic in a large soup and cook over medium heat.
- Add chicken stock and bring to a boil over high heat.
- Now add the green beans and tomato to the pot and cook for about 15 minutes.
- And add BBQ Sauce, shredded chicken, salt, and black pepper to the pot.
- Ladle the soup into serving bowls and top with shredded mozzarella cheese and cilantro to serve.

Grilled Salmon Soup

10 Servings

Preparation time: 25 minutes

Ingredients

- 6 cups Swiss chard, roughly chopped
- 4 Italian squash, chopped
- 2 garlic cloves, crushed
- 1 lemon, juiced
- Salt and black pepper, to taste
- 4 eggs
- 8 cups chicken broth
- 6 salmon fillets, chunked
- 4 tablespoons butter
- 2 cups parsley, chopped

Directions

- We have to make a chicken broth; now, put the chicken broth and garlic into a pot and bring to a boil.

- Add salmon, lemon juice, and butter into the pot and cook for about 10 minutes on medium heat.
- Now add Swiss chard, Italian squash, salt, and pepper and cook for about 10 minutes.
- Whisk eggs and add to the pot, stirring continuously.
- Garnish with parsley and serve.

Lightning Source UK Ltd.
Milton Keynes UK
UKHW020640220621
385951UK00004B/99